Grandma's Remedies

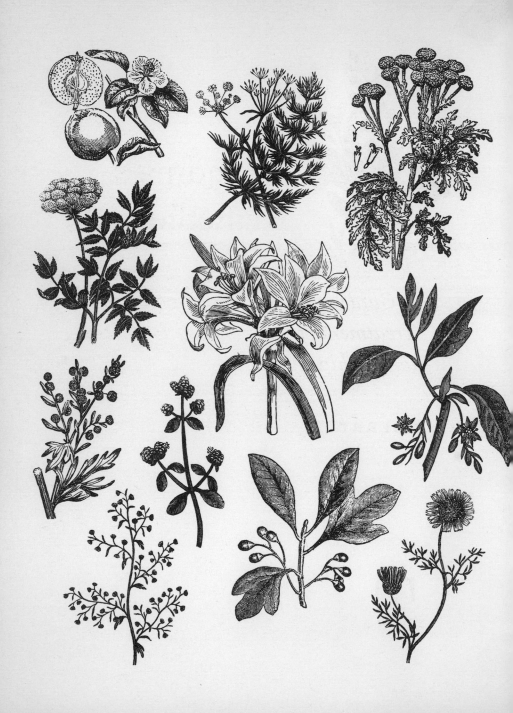

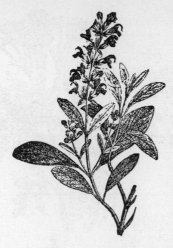

Grandma's Remedies

A Guide to Traditional Cures and Treatments from Mustard Poultices to Rosehip Syrup

CHERRY CHAPPELL

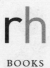

BOOKS

Published by Random House Books 2009

10 9 8 7 6 5 4 3 2 1

First published in Great Britain in 2009 by Random House Books
Random House, 20 Vauxhall Bridge Road, London SW1V 2SA

www.rbooks.co.uk

Addresses for companies within The Random House Group Limited can be found at:
www.randomhouse.co.uk/offices.htm

The Random House Group Limited Reg. No. 954009

A CIP catalogue record for this book is available from the British Library

ISBN 9781905211173

The information in this book has been compiled by way of general guidance on the specific
subjects addressed and is not a substitute, nor to be relied on, for medical, healthcare,
pharmaceutical or other professional advice. Please consult a professional practitioner before
changing, stopping or starting any medical treatment. The author and publishers disclaim,
as far as the law allows, any liability arising directly or indirectly from the use, or misuse,
of the information contained in this book.

The Random House Group Limited supports The Forest Stewardship Council (FSC),
the leading international forest certification organisation. All our titles that are printed on
Greenpeace approved FSC certified paper carry the FSC logo. Our paper procurement
policy can be found at www.rbooks.co.uk/environment

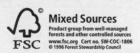

Mixed Sources
Product group from well-managed
forests and other controlled sources
www.fsc.org   Cert no. SW-COC-1806
© 1996 Forest Stewardship Council

Designed and typeset by Richard Marston
Printed and bound in Great Britain by Clays Ltd, St Ives plc

Contents

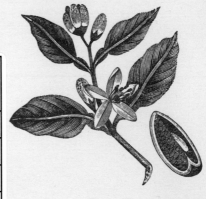

To Annie, Joan, Betty and Janet – and all the wise women who appear in these pages.

A short history of medicine

'Doctor, I have an earache.'

2000 BC: 'Hear, eat this root.'

AD 1000: 'That root is heathen. Hear, say this prayer.'

AD 1850: 'That prayer is superstition. Hear, drink this potion.'

AD 1940: 'That potion is snake oil. Hear, swallow this pill.'

AD 1985: 'That pill is ineffective. Hear, take this antibiotic.'

AD 2000: 'That antibiotic is artificial. Hear, take this root.'

Anon

Introduction

This book is an attempt to capture some of the healthcare practices and treatments that our grandmothers and those who came before them used for their own well-being and that of their families and communities. Many of the old remedies are both effective and inexpensive, and the recommendations – for example, advocating careful convalescence after illness – are often worth heeding. The main part of the text is an A–Z listing of remedies and advice gathered from all over the world. You will then find a section about the people, especially the women, who have contributed to our knowledge of how the human body functions and who, despite little encouragement and frequently blatant prejudice, practised and published their findings. The last part of the book is designed to help you follow in your grandmother's footsteps: to build your own home pharmacy, even to make a kitchen garden and to practise some of the methods that stood our forebears in such good stead.

However, this is not a 'herbal'. Instead it is a compendium of home or 'folk' remedies, many of which include the use of herbs, but also other plant materials, such as bark, tree flowers, seaweed, even minerals and what we normally consider to be foodstuffs, from eggs to onions. By and large, manufactured and branded remedies have not been included, although Vicks, Dolly Blue and bicarbonate of soda do make brief appearances.

The majority of these remedies have been used in living memory; some are still being taken or applied. They have lived on, often handed down orally, for countless years. In fact, it is impossible to know just how old some of these solutions are. Occasionally, in households where women were taught to read and write, favourite remedies were written in personal notebooks or in the back of cookery books. Often the remedies were jumbled up together with food recipes, domestic tips and hints, sayings and poems, and addresses. These books are fascinating and add to our knowledge of social history.

It has really been only in the last half-century that people have moved easily and regularly to different parts of the country or even different countries for education, career and retirement. Before that, communities were far more settled. In the 1800s one-third of the population worked on the land, although this figure had dropped to one-tenth by 1900. Transport – or lack of it – contributed to the isolation of many communities. Roads were often difficult and virtually impassable at certain times of the year, and travel was expensive. This continued until the railways were established. Even so, many women moved from their home area when they married, with the result that remedies and healthcare practices were circulated, and a number of remedies have become universally adopted.

By and large, remedies were concocted from what could be found locally. These were everyday, practical solutions to basic healthcare and first aid, and they were largely free from ritual and superstition

– although one or two myths did carry through. They were usually cost-effective, if not free, being developed and used by people, whether in a city or a rural area, for whom a doctor's fee was prohibitive in all but the direst need. Self-reliance was a necessity.

However, the well-to-do would self-administer too. Those in country areas would often have kitchen gardens where medicinal as well as culinary herbs were grown. Of course, the British also travelled throughout the world, as explorers and settlers, and they both took their know-how with them and brought back remedies they found in other parts of the world. Nowadays, the wonderful cultural mix found in Britain has added to the rich undercurrent of home medicine, with Ayurvedic and traditional Chinese herbs available on the high street.

Herbal myths

It is hard to know in common parlance when a plant can be considered a herb and when it is more properly a food. The botanical definition of a herb is a plant whose stem does not produce persistent, woody tissue and generally dies back at the end of the growing season, although some plants that have been long recognised as herbs are evergreen – rosemary, for example – and persist all year round. Some definitions also add that herbs are often aromatic and are used especially in medicine and food.

However, for many centuries herbs have been used not only as medicine – in the form of tinctures, infusions, teas, steam inhalants and so on – but also to flavour and preserve foods, sweeten rooms and fabrics, deter insects and vermin, and make cosmetics. In some cultures the dead were 'anointed' with herbs in the period before burial.

Herbs – and other plant material including bark, roots, leaves and mosses – have been the backbone of medical treatment for millennia. But, as the Royal College of Physicians acknowledges, the study of medicinal plants was 'sadly neglected by established medical professionals for many centuries. Apart from a few botanising enthusiasts in the sixteenth, seventeenth and eighteenth centuries, home-grown medicines were scorned or unknown by medical professionals, whose training was rigorously theoretical and classical. Even today, "green pharmacy" and alternative therapies are not fully utilised or recognised.'

Elsewhere in the world, such as in Africa, India and China, even now herbalism forms a part of traditional medicine that still outstrips the use of orthodox medicine, and in some European countries, notably in Germany and France, general practitioners receive training in herbalism and will prescribe herbal as well as allopathic drugs.

More recently, in this country, herbs have gained a reputation for their 'natural' qualities, and there is a worrying assumption that somehow they offer a gentler alternative to prescription drugs. The differences between the two must be examined.

It is true that many allopathic drugs are based on herbal substances. Estimates suggest that more than half of prescription drugs are derived from chemicals that were first identified in plants. For instance, some of the drugs used in the treatment of leukaemia and lymphatic cancer use vincristine, derived from periwinkle; the cancer drug paclitaxel is derived from the bark of the yew tree. Some of the larger pharmaceutical companies are currently investigating the old herbal remedies used by 'first nation' peoples in South American countries and Australia to see if they can be adapted into modern drugs.

The difference between pharmaceutical and herbal preparations is that conventional drugs are made from a particular element of the herb. A single active ingredient will be identified, extracted and then synthesised in a laboratory. Herbal preparations are made from a part of the whole plant – from the root, leaves, berries or flowers – and herbalists believe that the active constituents are balanced within the plant and are made more powerful by the various substances present.

We all know that many prescription drugs have side effects that affect some people more than others, but it is also true that particular herbs will suit some but not others.

Undoubtedly, herbal treatments are an alternative, and many have a long history of beneficial value, but they can be equally strong and, unless prescribed by a highly qualified and experienced practitioner, they can be every bit as dangerous as a wrongly prescribed conventional drug. Qualified herbalists will make sure that the herbal remedy is appropriate for the patient's particular constitution, age and condition and will prescribe only the best quality herbal preparation. Please read the Caution at the end of this introduction.

Belief and superstition

The elements that combine to produce healing are complex. Treatments that work for one patient may not work in the same way – or at all – for another, and many medical traditions across the world have recognised this. Orthodox medicine in the West tends to treat patients on the 'one size fits all' principle, offering predominantly drug therapies, surgery, physiotherapy and dialysis. Research into gene therapy may yield other elements.

Other traditions of medicine, those termed complementary, such as Ayurveda, the traditional medicine of India, or traditional Chinese medicine, look more deeply into a patient's individual constitution and any imbalances of energy. They pay close attention to the mind–body link and to diet and lifestyle, and may expect patients to adapt their lives as part of treatment.

However, there is one component of healing that all good healers will use: the patient's belief in their ability to be cured or, at least, to improve. Belief may come in different forms – belief in God or a higher power, belief in the healer or a belief in the treatment. Any and all of these appear to boost self-belief and the body's response.

The power of the mind–body link and the benefits of positive belief were identified by the most primitive societies, where healers were often priests, priestesses, shamans or conjurers. They surrounded their treatments with ritual, sometimes uplifting, sometimes gruesome, and in some societies they even used mind-enhancing or mind-altering drugs. The chanting of incantations, self-hypnosis and the use of talismans and animal or bird sacrifices were all designed to reinforce the healing process. Hippocrates, the father of medicine, who lived in the fifth century BC was the first person to split magic and medicine, insisting that disease was caused by mental and physical states of the body and environmental conditions, rather than demons and evil spirits. Despite this, the early Christian Church relied on religious ritual, including exorcism, for expelling various kinds of 'devils'. Many societies – including in Britain – up to the eighteenth century used elements of astrology for diagnosis and treatment.

In the West, however, science gradually turned orthodox medicine into something more mechanistic, with the body treated as a machine in which individual parts may fail, rather than an intricate meshing of mind–body responses, encompassing the physical, emotional and spiritual. Even so, most senior medical practitioners in orthodox medicine acknowledge the difference in outcomes when their patients have a positive mindset. This is seen clearly in many serious conditions and chronic diseases. An orthopaedic surgeon, who is very orthodox in his approach, admits that the personality of his patients is often the key to the quality of their lives. He is fond of quoting the example of two male patients both presenting with a similar condition – and extent – of osteoarthritis of the spine. One went home and told his wife: 'The doctor said it was a touch of arthritis so, that's it, I'm off to do a bit of gardening.' And so he did for many years afterwards. The other went home and said to his wife: 'The doctor said it's osteoarthritis so, that's it.' And he sat in his chair and very quickly became disabled.

Western doctors are also aware of the placebo effect. An example of this is when two groups of patients with similar conditions take part in a trial. One set will be given a drug, the other – without their knowledge – will be given a placebo or non-active substance. Only the researchers know which group has received the active drug. Often both groups will do equally well because all the participants believe that they are receiving a drug to cure their condition.

There are so many examples of the power of the mind over

matter: the Indian fakirs who rest on a bed of nails, the yogis who can raise and lower their own body temperature at will, the soldiers who fight on despite appalling injuries, the frail women who carry their children to safety – or the one who lifted a car off the body of her child – and those amazing souls who scorn diagnoses of terminal disease and overcome their health problems.

However, there comes a point where the unscrupulous can use the vulnerability and susceptibility of the unwell and turn belief into superstition in order to increase their own power. This then becomes a form of control and manipulation. Voodoo is a prime example: someone is told they will fall ill or die, and they promptly do so.

The fear of magic – of the unexplained, the unorthodox, the intuitive and all the general mess of human emotional states – is the strongest superstition of all. It led to the demise of the wise woman. In fact, the original definition of crone was a wise woman past childbearing age; a witch was a wise woman with special knowledge.

Despite all this, women have remained the primary healthcare workers in every community worldwide. Some of the remedies and practices in this book may initially appear a little unlikely, but it is extraordinary how many have a nugget of worth hidden within them. Instincts were sometimes spot on. Without scientific examination, some of the substances used – from chickweed to bee glue – have proved to be immensely effective. The stern determination of mothers and grandmothers everywhere that 'this will do the trick', 'this will cure you', seems to have done the rest. After all, we are all still here!

Measurements and quantities

In researching remedies for this book, I came across a number of different systems of measurement. Unsurprisingly, there were imperial weights (ounces and pounds, pints and quarts) as well as the metric forms (grams and litres). I also came across 'drachms' in some remedies dating from the 1800s or before, although it was a measure still in use in 1948 when Mrs E.W. Kirk wrote her *Tried Favourites Cookery Book*. See her mustard lotion remedy under Sprains (page 141). The dictionary definition of a drachm shows it to be fourteenth – century French from the Greek, meaning 'the number of coins one hand can hold'. In the UK a drachm – or dram – in the apothecaries' system was the equivalent of 60 grains or one-eighth of an ounce, which is 3.888 metric grams. A fluid dram was roughly the equivalent of one teaspoon – or just a smallish measure if being used to measure Scotch whisky.

'Grains' made a few appearances – for example in the 1739 remedy for dog bites – as did quantities by the pennyworth. For instance, a Mr Patterson gave Kate Fox of Aston, Oxfordshire, a remedy for whooping cough in which 2d (two pennyworth) of garlic was used. While one can translate a drachm into a modern equivalent, I suggest that weight by pennies was an imperfect science and probably relied on the judgement of the pharmacist – or in this case, the grocer.

The measurement system given in the original source has been left unchanged, with imperial or metric equivalents given in square brackets if appropriate. If you are trying any of these traditional remedies take great care when you convert them to your own preferred system, and remember to use either imperial or metric only, not a combination of the two.

Caution

Many of the remedies that appear in this book have not undergone formal clinical trials or have any scientific investigation behind them. The benefits of some herbs and herbal preparations are well documented, and their medicinal actions, energetics, uses and outcomes are known. So, too, are their contraindications – that is, those conditions and circumstances where their use is inappropriate. St John's wort (*Hypericum perforatum*) is a good example. It is widely prescribed in many parts of Europe as a safe anti-depressant, and there is research that shows it to be very effective. However, if it is combined with certain prescribed allopathic drugs, there may be detrimental side effects.

Most of the remedies and therapies selected here are not likely to cause serious side effects unless you are unfortunate enough to be sensitive or allergic to one of the ingredients or to be taking a prescription drug that causes a negative reaction.

We cannot take any responsibility for the effectiveness or outcomes of these remedies and therapies and strongly advise caution should you elect to try one or more of them. In the instances of herbal preparations, we recommend that you consult a qualified practitioner before experimenting. The National Institute of Medical Herbalists will help you find a qualified herbalist in your area via www.nimh.org.uk. There are also bodies, such as the Register of Chinese Herbal Medicine (www.herbmed@rchm.co.uk) and the

Ayurvedic Practitioners Association (www.apa.uk.com), which will put you in touch with their qualified practitioners.

In other instances, some of the remedies described in this book have been tested over centuries, and common sense suggests that they are perfectly safe to try. The application of a little honey to the inside of a nostril cracked by a cold or the use of radish juice to cure a verruca or wart should not hold too many perils. We leave it to the experience and wisdom of readers to differentiate.

It is also important to emphasise that if a condition persists, medical guidance should always be sought. Fevers, headaches and diarrhoea, for example, may be the symptoms of other underlying conditions. Our advice is, when in doubt, seek appropriate assistance.

A–Z of Remedies

Abscesses

a

Isaiah 38:21 records an instance from 2,400 years ago when figs were used to treat Hezekiah for his boils: 'For Isaiah had said, Let them take a lump of figs, and lay it for a plaster upon the boil.'

This remedy was echoed by Mrs Grieve in *A Modern Herbal* (1931), where she suggests that the figs are best roasted and split into two portions. The soft, pulpy interior may be applied as a smoothing poultice to treat gumboils and dental abscesses.

She also adds a recipe for green fig jam to aid well-being. It uses very juicy figs with the stalks removed but otherwise unpeeled. You then make a syrup with 8 oz [250 g] of sugar and ½ pint [300 ml] of water for each pound [500 g] of fruit. Placing the figs into the syrup, you cook them until the syrup pearls. You can add a stick of cinnamon and remove it before pouring the jam into suitable pots.

Figs for abscesses.

Acne

The bane of teenage life – and sometimes of later life too – acne has inspired numerous remedies, from treatments designed to cleanse the system to topical ointments using honey, which has antiseptic properties, or oatmeal, which is slightly abrasive. All the following remedies were suggested by teenagers, some of whom had heard about the treatments from their peers or parents, others who had tried everything and experimented. Now they have all moved on and have lovely complexions.

Acne is often thought to be linked to toxins in the system, and some youngsters recommended drinking litres of water and boosting their immune systems with vitamins in order to combat spots from within. There was even one suggestion of drinking dandelion tea, which has merit because dandelions are renowned for their cleansing qualities, particularly of the liver and urinary system.

People who preferred to attack the problem more directly would make up pastes and lotions for the affected areas. A number of these incorporated honey, including this exfoliant:

> *Mix one teaspoon of cinnamon into three tablespoons of honey.*
> *Use it as an exfoliant, that is, by gently working it into the affected areas. Leave for half an hour – or even overnight – and then wash off with warm water.*

Oatmeal and honey combined have also been used:

> *Make a paste of oatmeal softened with honey. Rub it into the affected areas and then leave for 20 minutes or so. Wash off with lots of cool water.*

There's a more elaborate version of this one too, combining the oatmeal with vinegar, raspberries, egg and salt:

Place the oatmeal in a small bowl, add about a tablespoon of salt, some raspberries, a splash of vinegar and an egg. Mix into a pink paste. Apply liberally, using it as a facial scrub. Leave for half an hour or until dry, then wash off with cold water.

An egg white makes an appearance in the following preparation, which also suggests it might help if you steam the face first:

Put hot water into a bowl, cover your head with a towel or cloth, lower your face over the bowl to about 4 inches from the surface of the water, capturing the steam within the towel. Close your eyes and wait for two or three minutes. This will open the pores of your skin. Mix two egg whites with a few drops of lemon. Whisk the mixture until it is frothy and apply as a mask to your skin. Allow it to dry then wash it off with cool water.

Sugar crystals, used in the following, have a slight abrasive quality and help remove dead skin, cleansing and opening the pores.

Wash the face with warm water but do not dry. Pour some granulated sugar into one hand. Pat it on to the affected areas of the skin and around the nose, chin and forehead. Rub gently in circular movements for three to four minutes. Rinse with warm water, followed by cold water.

For one persistent spot, Judy Townsend, who currently lives in Stratford-upon-Avon, suggests that a single raisin can help:

Place a raisin in boiling water to make it swell. Hold the raisin in place over the spot until it cools.

Several people recommended toothpaste, to be dabbed on a spot to dry it up. Another suggested salt worked into a paste and massaged into the face. This may sting if the skin is broken.

Ageing

Although we all know that there is no such thing as a fountain of youth, this hasn't stopped many people over the years seeking elixirs for longevity. Some were herbal, and the herb sage (*Salvia officinalis*) was particularly renowned, for example in the medieval medical school in Salerno, where doctors would quote: 'Why does the man in whose garden sage grows die?' To combat the symptoms of ageing this herb may have been combined with rosemary, credited with aiding memory, possibly by increasing the blood supply to the brain, or sweet marjoram, which helps protect against chills and reputedly boosts the elimination of wastes from the urinary system, so helping people with gout and arthritis.

An even older remedy is chywanaprash, a combination of herbs and spices, including cinnamon and cardamom, which are mixed with honey to make a rich jam. It was originally created to give the elderly sage Chywana the required virility to satisfy his young bride. It must have been successful because, even after 3,000 years, it remains in the Indian Ayurvedic tradition and is still readily available, although now it is more usually given to boost immunity and to aid convalescence.

A rather charming combination of anti-ageing herbs can be found in Act 4, Scene 3 of *The Winter's Tale* (*c*.1611) when Perdita makes a thoughtful posy for her middle-aged admirer, Polixenes, the king of Bohemia:

> *Here's flow'rs for you;*
> *Hot lavender, mints, savory, marjoram;*
> *The marigold, that goes to bed wi' th' sun,*
> *And with him rises weeping: these are flow'rs*
> *Of middle summer, and I think they are given*
> *To men of middle age.*

In the century after Shakespeare, the great herbalist Nicholas Culpeper (1616–54) listed all the qualities of these herbs: the aroma of mint was claimed to aid memory, lavender was a cure-all but specially useful to cure 'griefs and pains of the head', marjoram oil had the reputation of easing stiff joints, as, in a poultice, did savory, while marigolds strengthened the heart.

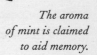

The aroma of mint is claimed to aid memory.

Anxiety

Anxiety is a state of apprehension and fearfulness that can become habitual or lead to panic attacks. Modern-day stress, with its overtones of burn-out and nervous exhaustion, is a close cousin and many of the remedies could be used for both unwelcome states.

Massage has been used since ancient times as a way of relaxing not only the body but also the mind, both in the East and the West.

It is interesting that massage is routinely prescribed in some countries, including France, for hypertension. Increasingly, masseurs are working in hospitals in the UK too. A back and shoulder massage, for instance, can effectively bring down blood pressure in cardiac patients if they are unable to take drugs. Ricky Clark-Monks from Chelsea uses a similar technique to help calm people who are having panic attacks, massaging their arms, using strokes from the shoulder to the hands. He believes that it pulls the energy down and away, literally stroking out the panic.

Yoga practitioners see the breath as the bridge between the mind and the body. Deep breathing can be a powerful therapy for panic attacks. When they are under stress, most people start to breathe in a shallow way at the very top of their lungs. It's no wonder people call the sensation 'breathlessness'. Consciously breathing slowly, using the sides and lower part of the lungs, is a classic way to gain control and calmness.

Sweet, milky drinks can also relieve anxiety, and there is scientific support for this claim. Milk contains an amino acid called tryptophan that stimulates the production of seratonin, which, in turn, calms the mind. Sugar releases insulin, which detracts the other amino acids, making tryptophan more effective.

See also Depression; Insomnia; Stress.

Arthritis see Osteoarthritis; Rheumatism

Asthma

The numbers of people with asthma are staggering: there are an estimated 200 million sufferers worldwide, with two million in Britain, including one in seven children.

The traditional French remedy for a severe attack is to drink two cups of strong black coffee. Unsurprising, perhaps, given how popular the drink is in France, but this is more than just a typical piece of Gallic insouciance. There have been substantial clinical studies on this practice, including one from Manitoba, Canada, of which the results were published in the *New England Journal of Medicine*. It confirms that caffeine relieves any bronchial obstruction, thereby easing and improving breathing. Coffee is, of course, a powerful stimulant for the nervous and cardio-vascular systems – some people find it too stimulating and experience palpitations. So even though this remedy has been shown to have some merit, it's certainly not a substitute for medicine but rather an emergency measure in the event of an attack, and it is especially not recommended for pregnant women.

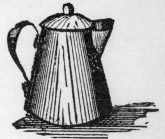

Coffee for asthma.

Other studies suggest that there are also beneficial effects from chocolate (again, two cups and again, only in emergencies). Because of its magnesium content chocolate is renowned as an anti-depressant too.

The French also believe in massage, and over the years French grandmothers have recommended one that uses garlic oil. It would not have smelled particularly attractive, but it may well have been efficacious following an attack.

*Place two cloves of garlic in 50 cl [17 fl oz] of olive oil. Apply
the mixture to the soles of the feet and at the base of the spine and
massage gently. Garlic is reputed to boost the body's defences.*

The practice of applying garlic to the soles of the feet has a long
pedigree. It's been used since Egyptian times to treat leprosy and
smallpox, and it was believed that, for best results, it needed to be
applied to the soles of the feet in a linen cloth, which would be
replaced regularly.

Garlic was also used internally as an asthma remedy. In her
Modern Herbal, which dates from 1931, Mrs Grieve gives two recipes
for syrup of garlic that she recommends not only for asthma but
also for hoarseness, coughs and breathing difficulties. The first uses
a quart of boiling water to which you add a pound of sliced fresh
garlic. The next step is to introduce sugar until the mixture is the
consistency of syrup. Vinegar and honey can then be added to taste.

An alternative is to boil garlic bulbs until they are soft, then add
an equal quantity of vinegar to the water in which the bulbs were
boiled. Again, you add sugar and boil the mixture down to make a
syrup. The bulbs are kept in the liquid. Mrs Grieve suggests taking
one or two bulbs and a little of the syrup every morning.

Pamela Jackson of Basingstoke remembers the herbaceous perennial hemp agrimony (*Eupatorium cannabinum*) being used for
asthma, though she can't vouch for its effectiveness. A gypsy used to
visit their home and told her grandmother to:

*dry the leaves of hemp agrimony, and then set light to them [pre-
sumably in a safe, fireproof bowl] so they smouldered. The treatment
was to inhale the fumes.*

An even older tradition is to use frankincense in the treatment of asthma and other respiratory complaints. Its distinctive aroma helps to slow down and regulate the breathing. Frankincense is a resin that comes from a small tree, *Boswellia thurifera*, which grows throughout Africa and in parts of the Middle East, particularly around the Red Sea. The tree's sap forms small peas of resin, which are burned to create the unique fragrance. Many of us will have first heard of frankincense in the story of the Nativity, where the three wise men bring gold, frankincense and myrrh as gifts for the baby Jesus. At that time, frankincense was highly prized as a holy perfume for use in religious rites. Indeed, 500 years earlier frankincense had been an important part of the annual tribute some subjects paid to the Persian emperor Darius the Great (*c*.548–486 BC).

Frankincense is also used in Ayurvedic medicine, the ancient health system of India, to treat a wide range of conditions. It is thought to be an anti-inflammatory and so is particularly useful for pain caused by cold and damp conditions or by swelling – in osteo- and rheumatoid arthritis, for example – and it is used to hasten the healing of wounds and broken bones. It also features in treatments for colitis, Crohn's disease, fibroids, cysts and painful periods. When it's not being pressed into service treating this wide range of ailments, it can also be used as an essential oil to open the mind.

Athlete's foot

A fungal infection, athlete's foot causes intense itching and cracked skin between the toes. It is a form of ringworm and is often picked up in public areas, such as changing rooms, gyms and swimming pools.

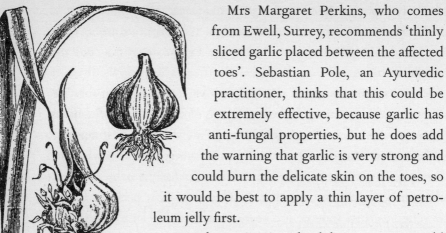

Mrs Margaret Perkins, who comes from Ewell, Surrey, recommends 'thinly sliced garlic placed between the affected toes'. Sebastian Pole, an Ayurvedic practitioner, thinks that this could be extremely effective, because garlic has anti-fungal properties, but he does add the warning that garlic is very strong and could burn the delicate skin on the toes, so it would be best to apply a thin layer of petroleum jelly first.

An alternative is calendula or pot marigold (*Calendula officinalis*), which probably came originally to Britain from India. It has been used for many centuries to treat various kinds of skin conditions, including burns, sunburn, inflammation, rashes, boils (see page 19) – as well as athlete's foot. Like garlic, it has anti-fungal properties, but it also has antiseptic and astringent qualities that can help if the affected areas are particularly sore. During the American Civil War doctors recognised its useful properties as they used the plant's leaves to staunch open wounds.

Garlic oil massage for asthma.

Here is a remedy for a pot marigold lotion suggested by Janet Mead of Coventry:

Place 4 oz [125 g] of fresh calendula flowers or 2 oz [50 g] of dried flowers in a large bowl. Cover with about 1 pint [600 ml] of boiling water. Allow to steep and to cool. Strain. Apply to the affected area using clean cotton wool. Cider vinegar can be added in equal parts where the skin is inflamed.

Not only is pot marigold useful for healing, it also has many uses in the kitchen. Its flowers can be used as a substitute for saffron in cooking when making rice or soup, and they are also a delightful addition to salads.

Herbal footbaths can be used when several toes or both feet are affected by athlete's foot. A strong infusion of the root of goldenseal (*Hydrastis canadensis*), a perennial herb in the buttercup family, is traditional in North America, as is the following mixture:

> *Take 10 oz [300 g] each of red clover, sage, calendula and agrimony. Add two treasons [2 pints/1.2 litres] of cider vinegar. Bathe the feet for half an hour, dry carefully and dust with powdered goldenseal root.*

Another approach is to massage the feet with an appropriate essential oil. Myrrh is especially good as it has anti-fungal properties. Mixing ten drops of myrrh essence with two tablespoons of vegetable oil produces a rub that is not only effective but also smells wonderful. My personal favourite, though, is essential oil of lavender, which is one of the few oils that you can safely use in an undiluted form directly on to the skin. A few drops applied with cotton wool when the itching starts always seems to do the trick for me. Lavender oil is both antibacterial and antiseptic and, of course, it also has a beautiful and calming scent.

Back pain

Given that back pain is such a common complaint in Britain, it is surprising that there are not more traditional therapies that might help ease it. Perhaps this can be put down to the fact that there are a number of different kinds of back pain: lumbago, where the pain is in the muscles and ligaments; slipped disc or sciatica, where the nerves are pinched; and inflammatory conditions, caused by rheumatism or ankylosing spondylitis. All are painful and incapacitating, but all require different types of treatment. Nowadays, many people find osteopathy, chiropractic and acupuncture useful, and there are qualified practitioners in most parts of the country.

When it comes to managing the pain at home, many people believe that heat is helpful in instances where there is any form of arthritis or muscle pain. A hot water bottle placed in an area of dull but persistent pain, for example, can offer some relief, while ice packs may help where there is inflammation. Sometimes alternating hot and cold compresses can ease the pain. A traditional method, called a fomentation, involved applying two towels, one wrung out with very hot water, the other with cold, alternately (see page 230).

People who are unfortunate enough to be struck with chronic back pain tend to develop ways of adapting their lives – the way they carry and lift objects, sit at work stations and so on – in order to avoid causing their particular pain. But when it does strike, a massage can help. Here is a massage preparation from a 'receipt book' dating from 1687, which originally belonged to a woman called Mary Goodson but is now in the possession of the Royal College of Physicians.

For payne of the back or boddy
    Take the oyle of Angelica and Camomile
and elder flowers, all oyles mixed together,
Annoynte the place with your warme hands.

Bedsores

Bedsores are nasty lesions that can occur when someone is bedridden or confined to a wheelchair for long periods. One of my correspondents for this book, Catherine Gould, had a great-grandmother called Clara 'Kate' Fox, who kept a book of her handwritten 'receipts' – the old term for remedies and recipes – probably in the 1860s or 1870s. As with so many of these books, the notes covered all kinds of household concerns, so that remedies for whooping cough or burns were listed alongside those for making a furniture polish or exterminating ants. For bedsores, she noted:

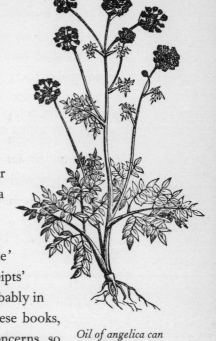

Oil of angelica can be combined with other herbs to treat back pain.

> *Equal parts of eau-de-Cologne and Brandy and the two propor-*
> *tions of best olive oil, well mixed together and applied. Zinc powder*
> *sprinkled on is also very healing.*

A century later Jean Rogerson, a nurse at the former Bolton District Hospital, used methylated spirits:

> *In the 1960s and 1970s we would wash bedridden patients with*
> *soap and water, concentrating on their heels, elbows, shoulders, back*

*and bottom, then dry them off. We would put methylated spirits
on the palms of our hands and massage it in to toughen the skin
so bedsores were less likely to form. The massage also encouraged
blood flow.*

Another former nurse, now married to a GP, suggests a remedy that
is very similar to one for nappy rash (see page 123).

*Turn your patient over. Apply egg white to the sores. Cover them
completely and allow the egg white to dry. Sometimes we would use a
blast of oxygen to help the drying!*

In her *Tried Favourites Cookery Book* (1948) Mrs Kirk also suggested using an egg white preparation to prevent 'galling' in people
who were confined to bed:

*The white of an egg, beaten to a strong froth, then drop in gradu-
ally whilst you are beating two teaspoons of spirits of wine; put it into
a bottle, and apply occasionally with a feather.*

While I was gathering material for this book I noticed that egg
whites frequently cropped up in traditional remedies dealing with
spots or lesions, but it is difficult to uncover any scientific basis for
this. Peter Homan of the Royal Pharmaceutical Society of Great
Britain, who has managed to solve several of the book's mysteries,
unfortunately drew a blank with egg whites. Having been through
a whole range of historical sources, Peter found the following uses
for egg white: diarrhoea in infants, metallic – for example mercury
– poisoning; nutrition and clarification, such as in wine-making.
However, he couldn't find any mention of egg whites to treat sores
or any explanation of their efficacy.

Bee stings

In the mid-nineteenth century a company called William Edge & Sons at Backbarrow, Cumbria, began to manufacture a synthetic blue ultramarine 'for gleaming whites on washday'. The factory – and the product – became known as 'Dolly Blue', probably stemming from the names of Victorian laundry equipment: the dolly tub was filled with hot water for laundry, and the dolly peg, with its four or five legs, was used to move the clothes around in the tub. The product was made from china clay, caustic soda, sulphur and other substances ground together and baked, and it came in the form either of a large block of blue with a stick in it, or a small block held in a muslin bag that would be added to washing. Dolly Blue is no longer available – production ceased around 1981 – but you can find a similar product in the USA called Bluette or Mrs Stewart's Bluing.

As well as whitening whites, Dolly Blue was used to treat bee stings, and this remedy was renowned not only in Britain but also in Australia and New Zealand. The advice was: 'Blue bag for bees, vinegar for wasps.' Sylvia Coppen-Gardner from Gloucester mentioned that a blue bag was used not only for stung humans but also on one memorable occasion when a bee stung her dog's nose.

Other equally effective remedies include this one, supplied by Betty Browning of Coventry, which uses raw onion:

> *Ensure that the sting is fully removed. Cut an onion in half and apply the freshly cut side directly over the puncture mark to reduce swelling and pain.*

An Australian friend recalls the following remedy:

> *Make a paste of baking soda by adding a few drops of water.*
> *Apply this to neutralise the sting. Then apply a drop of lavender oil*
> *directly on to the site of the sting to relieve itching or pain.*

Blood cleansing and cooling

Norris Winstone of Norwich, who at the time of writing is
ninety-four, recalls his grandmother, Grannie Bub, making special
sandwiches of nasturtium, dandelion leaves and watercress for the
children in the family in order to 'cleanse the blood'. There's a lot
of nutritional value in this remedy. Nasturtium (*Tropaeolum*) is a
great source of vitamin C, and the leaves of dandelions (*Taraxacum
officinale*) have been proved to stimulate bile production in the liver.
But the most important ingredient is probably watercress, which is
rich in iron, potassium, calcium, sulphur and phosphorous, as well
as a number of vitamins – its vitamin C levels are particularly high.
A member of the Cruciferae family – which includes cabbages,
Brussels sprouts, broccoli, kale, turnip and horseradish – watercress
is actually related to nasturtium, which also contains potassium and
a mustard oil that gives both their peppery 'bite'. In *Superfoods*
Michael van Straten and Barbara Griggs suggest that watercress is
beneficial to the digestive system and is a good source of iodine,
which is useful for low thyroid activity.

In about 400 BC Hippocrates, the father of medicine, is supposed
to have founded his first hospital beside a stream so that he could
have watercress beds close by to boost his patients' recovery. It is

also said that the Greek general Xenophon encouraged his soldiers to eat it before battle to increase their vigour. Its properties are still valued. In 2008 the Watercress Alliance funded a research project at the University of Southampton to investigate the anti-cancer properties of watercress, particularly in relation to breast cancer.

Mention brimstone and treacle and most people think of Dennis Potter's 1976 play. In fact, brimstone and treacle was originally a Victorian remedy. There's a reference to it in Charles Dickens's *Nicholas Nickleby* (1838–9):

> *Mrs Squeers stood at one of the desks, presiding over an immense basin of brimstone and treacle, of which delicious compound she administered a large instalment to each boy in succession: using for the purpose a common wooden spoon, which might have been originally manufactured for some gigantic top, and which widened every young gentleman's mouth considerably: they being all obliged, under heavy corporal penalties, to take in the whole of the bowl at a gasp.*

Watercress for cleansing the blood.

It is also remembered by Marjorie Goodman from Colchester, who says that a tablespoon of brimstone and treacle was given to her to 'cool the blood' every spring during her childhood in the 1920s. It consisted of yellow sulphur powder mixed into treacle – or golden syrup – and, apparently, it was not unpleasant.

Christine Fletcher from Broughton, Hampshire, recalls how her father also took brimstone and treacle once a week, but in this instance it was to 'keep regular'.

The herb traditionally associated with both cleansing and 'thinning' the blood is red clover (*Trifolium pratense*). It is a diuretic and a mild laxative, but it is credited with anti-viral and anti-fungal properties too. It is still used by modern herbalists, particularly to help women's problems, such as heavy or painful periods or following the menopause. In homeopathy it is used for, among other conditions, cancer, coughs and throat complaints, skin conditions and tension headaches.

See also Immune system.

Boils

A number of people remember milk bottles being used to 'draw' a boil or carbuncle. Norman Drysdale from Glasgow recalls developing a nasty boil on his neck while he was serving in the army in the 1950s:

> *One of the medics heated an empty milk bottle and put the mouth of it over the boil. The heat and the vacuum of air drew the pus out of the boil, just sucked it out.*

However, the greatest caution must be used here. This method may be effective, but it is very drastic and must never be used on the face as it may lead to scarring.

The other popular remedy was to make up a poultice or a hot compress. See page 228 for making poultices, which have many applications, from easing muscle pain to warming a chilled patient.

Three types of poultice, however, have been recommended especially for treating boils. In the north Devon WI cookbook, Mrs E.C. Hopper from Alwington suggests a baked onion poultice:

> Bake a piece of onion (half an onion can be baked in a tin on the hob; no need to use the oven). Take out an inner ring and cover the affected part. Bandage to keep it in place, renew the poultice night and morning.

Mrs Shirley Reynolds from the Isle of Wight recalls a poultice made with bread and vinegar that would be used to draw out the pus from boils and carbuncles:

> Boil bread and vinegar together and place on a clean cloth such as white cotton sheeting. Squeeze out excess moisture, making the mulch into a pad. Place the pad over the infected area and cover with a piece of waterproof material, and then fix with plasters or bandages. Renew the pad every few hours, as it cools, until the wound is clear of infection and matter.

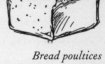

Bread poultices
for boils.

The herbalist and author Michael van Straten opts for pot marigold (*Calendula officinalis*):

> Make a poultice from the petals from marigold flowers, which have both antiseptic and anti-fungal properties, to draw a boil or soothe painful infection.

A different solution comes from another famous herbalist, Mrs Grieve (1931), who advocated the use of a lotion made from elderflowers by pouring water on dried blossoms:

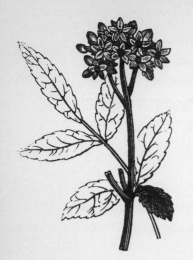

*Elderflower lotion
for boils.*

*Mix 2½ drachms of elder flowers to 1 quart
[2 pints/1.2 litres] of boiling water, infuse for one
hour and then strain.*

For people who regularly experienced boils,
Robert McElhinney from Horn Head in County
Donegal recalls that the remedy was bog bean,
also known as buckbean and marsh trefoil
(*Menyanthes trifoliata*), which, as the common
name suggests, grows in boggy land. To treat
boils bog beans were boiled in water, strained
and then the liquid was taken daily by the glass
in order to clean the blood. Robert also recalls that the
whole plant, including the roots, was sometimes boiled
to make a blood-cleansing drink, while a tea could be made from the
dried leaves to help with headaches and migraine.

Bronchitis

A mustard plaster can be very effective in treating chest conditions,
even if it does sound the stuff of Victorian nightmares. Here is the
remedy that Eileen Fardon's grandmother, Bessie Bloomfield, used:

*1 oz [25 g] of dry mustard
Teaspoon of plain flour*

*Mix to a paste with vinegar. Spread on a rag or piece of muslin
and make a sandwich of it: material/mustard paste/material. Keep
on the chest no longer than 10 minutes, otherwise it will burn.*

As in treatments for coughs and chesty colds, there was a widely held belief that the chest should be covered with various kinds of grease – goose fat, for instance – and then with brown paper or some form of dense fabric or wadding. It acted as a kind of lagging that helped the body retain its own heat. Nancy Lowther of Ramsgate used best goose fat as a 'plastering' for her son Peter, who, although hating the smell, admitted that he found it soothing. Shirley Reynolds from Yarmouth on the Isle of Wight remembers a large piece of flannel being soaked in olive oil and turpentine and fastened across the patient's 'tight' chest. She says: 'The fumes were inhaled and it helped to ease the pain and coughing.'

Inhalants, of course, were often used as remedies on their own. Herbs such as eucalyptus, an evergreen tree that is native to Australia, and hyssop (*Hyssopus*), a member, like mint, of the Labiatae family, were found to be helpful in relieving congestion. To inhale, simply put a few drops of essence on a paper towel or add them to a bowl of hot water.

But inhalants and rubs are certainly not for everyone, and in some cases a more gentle solution was preferred. Take this recipe for turnip syrup:

> *Slice a turnip, place it in a dish and cover with brown sugar. Leave overnight. Drink it the following morning to help expel the phlegm.*

An alternative was to use liquorice (*Glycyrrhiza glabra*), which has a long history as a medicinal plant. Mentioned by Roman writers, including the great healer Dioscorides, it was used in various parts of Europe during the Middle Ages and was cultivated in England from about 1562. According to Mrs Grieve in her *Modern Herbal* (1931) it could be used for coughs and chest complaints, notably bronchitis. She recommended making an infusion by boiling 1 oz (25 g) of peeled and bruised liquorice with 1 pint (600 ml) of water for a few minutes. The sweetness in liquorice comes from the compound glycyrrhizin, which is supposedly fifty times stronger than sugar and has been shown by recent Japanese studies to have anti-viral properties.

See also Colds (chesty).

Bruises

In Act 3, Scene 1 of *Love's Labour's Lost* (*c.*1594) Costard, the clown, takes a tumble and damages his shin and calls for plantain from the pageboy, Moth: 'O! sir, plantain, a plain plantain ... no salve, sir, but a plantain.'

Plantain (*Plantago*) is found throughout Europe, North America and Asia, but it appears to have been used in medicine for the first time in China during the Han Dynasty (206 BC–AD 24). The seeds are still used today to make commercial laxatives, and it has been suggested that it improves some forms of IBS (Irritable Bowel Syndrome). Its leaves – as Costard knew – can also be used externally to treat bruises and to stop bleeding.

Seventeenth-century herbalist Nicholas Culpeper rated plantain highly, suggesting many uses for it including the following:

> *The juice of the Plantain clarified and drank for divers days together, either of itself, or in other drink, prevails wonderfully against all torments or excoriations in the intestines and bowels, helps*

the distillations of rheum in the head, and stays all matters of fluxes, even women's courses, when they flow too abundantly.

He also recommended it for consumption, lung ulcers and coughs, for dropsy and yellow jaundice; taken in water to help sore eyes and painful ears; for inflammation of the skin, scalds, mouth ulcers, gout, snake and dog bites, and pain from dislocated joints:

> *One Part of Plantain water, and two parts of the brine of powdered beef, boiled together and clarified, is a most sure remedy to heal all spreading scabs or itch in the head and body, all manner of tetters, ring-worms, the shingles, and all other running and fretting sores. Briefly the Plantains are singularly good wound herbs, to heal fresh or old wounds, either inward or outward.*

Barbara Hawkins from Brighton is now in her eighties, and in her youth she enjoyed visiting her grandmother, Eliza Baker, in Seaford, Sussex. She remembers that if ever she fell over, knocked or bruised herself, her grandmother would treat the sore places with a lotion made from quince pips and brandy. Barbara believes her grandmother made the lotion herself, probably using quinces from her grandfather's allotment. 'I loved the smell of it. The brandy always reminded me of Christmas, with the brandy on the pudding,' Barbara says.

Plantain for bruises.

Witch hazel (*Hamamelis*) is another standard remedy, offered here by Jean Rogerson, a nurse at the former Bolton District General Hospital:

> *Apply witch hazel to the site even before the bruising has had a chance to come out; it seems to stop the black blood from forming. Don't use it on broken skin though.*

Witch hazel originated in North America and was used by Native Americans who recognised its astringent qualities and used it to treat varicose veins, sprains, burns and inflammations as well as bruises. There are also some studies that show it has anti-inflammatory properties.

Burns (minor)

The best immediate treatment for a minor burn is to hold the affected area under cold running water. You can also put ice on to the area for a short time to take the heat out of the skin.

There are many people who have used honey on small burns, perhaps because it is soothing and has antiseptic qualities. Another more unusual – but recurring – recommendation is for raw grated potato. Valerie Witts's mother, Bessie Jones, who lived in Aylesbury, followed this recipe:

> *Grate a potato and place it on a burn to relieve the pain. When the potato turned brown or the pain returned, repeat the process.*

A more elaborate potato paste, using much the same principle, comes from Martha Mlinaris in Shepton Mallet, Somerset:

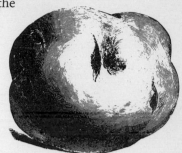

> *Grate raw potato into a bowl. Add a*
> *pinch of salt. Add some flour to make*
> *a paste. Spread the paste gently on to*
> *the burnt area and hold in place with a*
> *cloth. It will draw the heat out of the burn.*
> *As the paste gets hot, take it off and replace*
> *with fresh cold paste. Keep changing the paste*
> *as it heats up. When the burn is better, keep it covered.*

Potato will soothe burns.

She stresses that it is important not to use this remedy on burns if the skin is broken.

Some people recommend putting butter on a burn, but only when the skin is not broken. In France it is believed that butter or oils should not be used on their own because they are not sterile. They prefer to take an egg yolk, add a little butter, then place the mixture on some gauze before holding it in position with a bandage. They will also use a beaten egg white applied on gauze to the affected area to take away the pain.

Another French remedy is to cut an onion and apply it directly to a small burn. This will sting and so takes courage. The remedy can be improved if you add a pinch of salt, but this takes even more courage!

Burns or scalds (where the skin is broken)

Catherine Gould found this 'receipt' in a personal notebook belonging to her great-grandmother Kate Fox from Aston in Oxfordshire.

> *Slake some lime with cold water, when it has stood some time pour carefully off and mix lime water with an equal quantity of linseed oil. Shake well until as thick as cream.*

This is followed by a note: 'If put in a bottle and tightly sealed, it will keep for years.' According to Peter Homan of the Royal Pharmaceutical Society of Great Britain, the lime water mentioned here is probably a solution of calcium hydroxide, which was used internally as an antacid and externally for its antiseptic and cooling properties.

In Powys there is also mention of 'lime' in this remedy for 'a violent burn or scald when the skin is off', dating from 1891.

> *A Lump of hot Lime put into cold Spring water, mix as much sweet oil as will make an emulsion with it and apply it.*

Chickenpox

One of the 'standard' childhood diseases, chickenpox is rare but can be a very serious condition in adults. After an incubation period, a mild fever develops, and this is followed by an itchy rash. Watery liquid forms in blisters that burst and form scabs. When I was a child, in the 1950s and 1960s, mothers would cut their children's nails as short as possible so they were unable to scratch the scabs and cause scarring.

There are a number of herbs that soothe the skin and so relieve the itching, among them sweet violet, rose (as a water) and camomile. You will find an infusion under Skin diseases that uses camomile with mallow and lemon verbena.

Chilblains

Onions seem to have some effect on chilblains, and they crop up in a number of old remedies. Eighty-nine-year-old Rhoda Old from Cornwall recalls a remedy given to her by a gypsy to be used only on chilblains where the skin is unbroken:

> Cut a raw onion in half and dip one half into salt and rub it briskly into the affected area.

A similar remedy was suggested by a member of Littleton WI in Cheshire.

Marina Bruce in Peterborough suffered every year from what she describes as 'horrendous chilblains', which her grandmother, Margaret Isbister, who came from Fetlar, Shetland, would treat:

Chop raw onions, apply liberally over the toes, securing them with a bandage and then with a sock overnight.

Marina reports: 'It did relieve the itching and swelling and much to my amazement my bed never smelt of onions.' Marina adds that recently she has started to get chilblains again but has decided not to use this method in case it 'perfumes' her bed.

Kate Fox from Aston, Oxfordshire, described the following ointment for 'broken chilblains' in her notebook, dated (it is believed) from 1860–70.

Take 7½ oz [220 g] yellow wax, 1 pint [600 ml] olive oil, place in a jar [and] stand in a pan of boiling water and thoroughly melt. While cooling, stir in 7½ oz [220 g] prepared calamine. Spread on to linen and bind up. [It is] healing and takes out inflammation.

In Wales, Powys in particular, there is a different version of this wax and oil remedy. This handwritten 'receipt' is displayed on pages of herbal remedies from an interesting website, www.day-in-the-life.powys.org.uk, which explores life in Powys in 1891 and compares it with the present day:

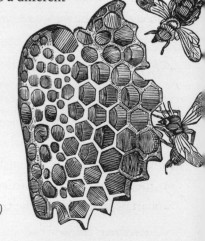

1 pint [600 ml] sweet oil
3 oz Venice [75 g] turpentine
1 lb [500 g] Hogs Lard (without salt)
3 oz [75 g] Bees Wax

Beeswax for chilblains

Put all into a pipkin or stone jar over a slow fire and stir it with
a wooden spoon till the Bees Wax is all melted and the ingredients
begin to simmer.

Another remedy sounds a bit eye-watering until you work through the logic: it is to bathe the affected area with urine. Jennifer Clifton from Folkestone tells of how one of her older sisters would suffer terribly as a child and the remedy was to 'pee in a pot and sit with your feet in it'. Malcolm Bean in north London received the same advice: 'My mother taught me to bathe chilblains in my own urine. This hardens the skin. It's a remedy that has been known since antiquity. After all, urine is used in tanning leather throughout the world.' Rowers, such as Christopher from north London who has rowed at the Henley Regatta, use the same method to harden the skin on their hands. More fragrant – though perhaps a touch less manly – solutions would be to massage areas, particularly where there is pain and itching, with lavender and marjoram.

Chills

Many a Scot will tell you that the very best remedy for spring, autumn or winter chills is the traditional hot toddy. At its most basic, this is a combination of whisky and hot water, and it is drunk to bring out a sweat and diminish any fever. There are many variations on the recipe, but this particularly delicious one came from Anne Stobart, a medical herbalist from Devon.

1 piece root ginger
2 teaspoons caraway seed

1 bottle of whisky

Grated zest and juice of one lemon

8 oz [250 g] of large fat raisins

> *Bruise the ginger and caraway seeds and place them in a wide-necked jar with all the other ingredients. Seal and leave for three weeks, shaking the jar daily, then strain and rebottle.*

As Anne explains: 'Drunk by itself or with hot water, this toddy is said to cure everything from an impending cold to seasickness. However, it is best used as a deterrent because alcohol wastes vitamin C, which is needed to fight off a cold. Flu or colds benefit from a simpler version of fresh ginger (sliced), lemon juice, honey and cinnamon with boiling water poured on and stirred well. Deliciously warming.' Ah, but does it have the kick?

Frances Wilkins from Habrough in northeast Lincolnshire offers what she describes as a lovely tummy warmer: 'a few drops of tincture of lavender on a lump of sugar.'

Choking

If something has 'gone down the wrong way' the universal solution is a swift slap on the back to dislodge the blockage. However, when the choking is caused by fish bones or small, pointed objects sticking in the throat a more subtle approach may be needed. In her *Tried Favourites Cookery Book* (1948) Mrs Kirk recommends:

> *Fluids should not be given, but a dry diet of bread, thick porridge, pudding or mashed potatoes, which will carry the object through the body. To remove a fish bone from the throat, suck a lemon which*

dissolves parts of the bone, and makes it quite flexible. Another way
is to swallow a raw egg immediately.

Of course, if this should fail, professional medical help should be
sought.

Cholera

It is easy to forget how many diseases our grandmothers lived in
fear of but that we now are able to disregard. Many have been all
but eradicated in the West, although sadly some are still prevalent in developing countries. Our grandmothers dreaded smallpox,
diphtheria, typhus, tuberculosis, polio, leprosy and cholera. Mary
Seacole (see pages 199–202) gained her reputation as a herbal
healer because of her success in treating cholera. In her biography
Wonderful Adventures of Mrs Seacole in Many Lands, written in 1857,
she describes the treatment she administered during an outbreak in
Cruces in Panama:

> *Another patient, a girl, I rubbed over with warm oil, camphor*
> *and spirits of wine. Above all, I never neglected to apply mustard*
> *poultices to the stomach, spine and neck, and particularly to keep*
> *my patient warm about the region of the heart. Nor did I relax my*
> *care when the disease passed by, for danger did not cease when the*
> *great foe was beaten off. The patient was left prostrate; strengthening*
> *medicines had to be given cautiously, for fever, often of the brain,*
> *would follow … few constitutions permitted the use of exactly the*
> *same remedies, and that the course of treatment which saved one*
> *man would, if persisted in, have very likely killed his brother.*

Mary Seacole employed a battery of treatments to deal with cholera, including mustard poultices and plasters, sugar of lead, cinnamon water and mercury. Sadly, she only left scant details of the recipes she used, but Helen Rappaport, author of *No Place for Ladies: The Untold Story of Women in the Crimean War*, has done some research into what would have been used and found some useful information in Martindale's *Pharmacopoeia*, first published in 1883. She suggests that mustard plasters would have been made of mashed mustard seeds that had been made into a paste and applied to the skin. The treated area would then have been massaged to improve the blood circulation and to warm it up. They would have been particularly effective in easing stiffness of joints, particularly in the neck and spine and in easing symptoms like cramps. Interestingly, there's a record of Hippocrates using a mustard poultice as an antidote to scorpion bites. They are still used in some European countries – France, German and Italy – for drawing infection, and on the Faroe Islands people have been known to place them on the cheek to alleviate the pain of toothache.

Mary Seacole was born in Jamaica, and cinnamon was a traditional part of that country's medicine. She mentions boiling the bark in water, and giving the liquid to her patients. Cinnamon is an astringent, but it's also used as a carminative (to relieve flatulence) and in the treatment of diarrhoea and mild gastro-intestinal disorders as well as respiratory conditions.

Cinnamon is an astringent.

Sugar of lead is another name for lead acetate, which can be poisonous and so would normally have been applied externally. If taken internally it would act as a purgative, and this is how Mary seems to have used it, adding 10 grains to a pint (600 ml) of water and giving the patient a tablespoonful every quarter of an hour.

Another poison that Mary thankfully applied externally was mercury, and other records show the use of the metal at this time as a treatment for syphilis and chronic skin diseases. Because it is extremely dangerous, the medical use of mercury had been more or less abandoned in Britain by the 1950s.

Kate Fox from Aston, Oxfordshire, wrote in her personal notebook in the mid-nineteenth century a remedy for the prevention of cholera:

> *A solution of 7½ grains citric acid to 1 quart [2 pints/1.2 litres] of water. This tends to destroy bacillus of cholera. If strength of solution is raised to 14 grains to 1 quart it will also destroy the bacillus of typhoid.*

Cholesterol

Our grandmothers did not have remedies specifically for high cholesterol simply because they were not aware of its existence. Establishing cholesterol levels requires a particular kind of blood test, which obviously would not have been available then. It's also probable that high cholesterol was not such a problem before the era of processed foods and fast-food chains. The type of life our grandmothers led may well have kept levels in check: they tended to eat locally grown or home produce when it was in season and to get plenty of physical exercise.

The Mediterranean diet seems to be particularly appropriate for people with high cholesterol, and Crete has the reputation for having the healthiest traditional diet: plenty of fish, virgin olive oil, locally grown vegetables, fruit and herbs. Olives are a natural antioxidant, and it is believed that they may help to lower cholesterol levels.

Recent experiments have also shown that raw onions may help reduce cholesterol by boosting levels of high-density lipoproteins, the molecules that clear cholesterol away from the walls of the arteries.

Cold and chapped hands

The famous Italian cook Antonio Carluccio describes how his mother used to boil chestnuts for her sons before they went to school, not just to eat, but so they could put them in their pockets and keep their hands warm on the journey to their classes. This must have helped prevent Antonio and his brother from getting chapped hands, which can be extremely painful. There are a number of traditional preparations that can help, including this one recorded by Marjorie Carwell, who was born in 1843 and who worked in service in Scotland throughout her life. 'Put a large teaspoon of honey into the water for washing your hands,' and after washing, apply camphor cream. The recipe uses spermaceti, a waxy, oily substance that comes from the head of sperm whales.

Gradually melt together 10 oz [300 g] of lard, 1 oz [25 g] of spermichetti, ½ oz [15 g] of camphor and ½ oz [15 g] of white wax.

Marjorie's collection of remedies from the nineteenth century was found first by her grandson and later by her granddaughter, Anne Bisset.

Also to avoid chapped hands, Mrs Kirk, who wrote the *Tried Favourites Cookery Book* in 1948, added this remedy in a section on 'useful information'.

> *Take common starch and grind it with a knife until it is reduced to the finest powder, put it in a clean tin box, so as to have it continually at hand for use. After washing your hands, rinse them thoroughly in clean water, wipe them, and while they are yet still damp rub a pinch of starch over them, covering the whole surface.*

She adds that 'the effect is magical and that the rough, smarting skin is cooled and healed'. To cure chaps she suggested:

> *Take an equal quantity of pure sweet oil and glycerine. Shake well before using. Pure glycerine without the admixture of oil is not to be recommended. A piece of mutton suet, melted in the oven, will be found very good for the hands.*

Cold sores on the lips

Unlike mouth cankers, which tend to be singular and inside the mouth, cold sores (lip herpes) usually take the form of a rash of small blisters clustered around one major site on the lips. They can be treated with propolis, a product of bees that is often called bee glue. Worker bees collect the resin from various kinds of buds and tree barks and use it to fill the cracks in the walls of the hive. It is largely resin but also contains elements of wax and pollen. According to *The Oxford Book of Health Foods*, there have been a number of scientific investigations into the efficacy of propolis, particularly in eastern Europe. The results indicate that extracts from propolis were effective against various bacteria, including *Mycrobacterium tuberculosis*, against the fungi involved in skin infections and also against the types of virus involved in colds and flu. Carola Augustin from Vienna recommends propolis for cold sores:

> *As soon as the first symptoms are detected, either put honey or propolis (bee glue) on the affected part of the lip. Keep the sore dry and apply the honey or propolis as often as possible.*

Carola has found that honey and propolis reduce the duration of the lip infection by half and, if applied early enough, can even hinder the emergence of the blister.

Vinegar is frequently mentioned as being useful in treating a cold sore, and another suggestion is toothpaste: 'Gently smoothe thick toothpaste on to the blister to help to dry it.'

Here is a recipe for an ointment with an unknown provenance but that seems like a delightful treatment for cold sores or for chapped skin:

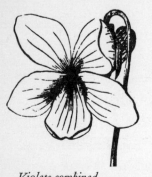

Violets combined with other ingredients for cold sores.

> *Combine 2 tablespoons of finely chopped fresh sage leaves with 2 tablespoons of sweet violets and 4 tablespoons of almond oil and pour them into a glass bottle. Stopper it tightly and leave it in a warm atmosphere for at least four weeks, agitating it daily. Strain before use. Melt together a further 4 tablespoons of almond oil and tablespoons of beeswax (you can*

use a bain-marie or container within a large saucepan of water) and
add the herbal liquid to it. Beat until it cools. Stopper it tightly. Store
in a cool place.

Lavender is one of the few essential oils that can be applied safely direct to the skin, and many people believe that a drop of lavender, which has antiseptic properties, should be applied to the blister of a cold sore to soothe and speed healing, and reduce the likelihood of scarring.

Colds

'Starve a fever, feed a cold,' runs the old adage. This makes sense, if only because with a high fever no one feels like eating anyway. And you may not taste much if you have a heavy cold, but you will feel less depleted if you take in nourishing foods. In my childhood home dairy products – milk, cheese and butter – were banned at the first sign of a cold on the grounds that they tend to encourage the production of mucus. I have since discovered that this is a tenet of both Ayurvedic (traditional Indian) medicine and traditional Chinese herbal medicine.

There are literally dozens of remedies to alleviate the misery of colds. Steam vapours were popular at one time, and in the 1950s and 1960s they often included a touch of eucalyptus oil, a traditional medicine of Australian Aborigines whose use of the tree probably dates back many thousands of years:

Fill a shallow bowl with hot water and add a drop or two of
eucalyptus oil. Drape a towel over your head. Lean over the bowl,

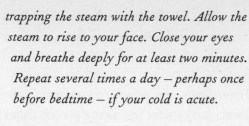

trapping the steam with the towel. Allow the steam to rise to your face. Close your eyes and breathe deeply for at least two minutes. Repeat several times a day – perhaps once before bedtime – if your cold is acute.

A useful remedy was gathered from Carola Augustin from Vienna for that stage in a cold when the inside of your nose becomes cracked and sore. She suggests that you reach for the honey.

Put a little on to your little finger and gently wipe the inside of your nose. Honey has antiseptic as well as calming properties that will benefit your nose and, by breathing it in, your sinuses too.

Eucalyptus inhalants for colds.

A number of older people remember being given blackcurrant jam, made into a syrup-like tea.

Take a good heaped tablespoon of blackcurrant jam and pour hot water over it.

Enid Troubridge of Godalming was given this remedy when she was a child, but she is unsure how effective the remedy was, although obviously it was a source of vitamin C. Whatever the health benefits may have been, she says that it tasted delicious.

An interesting suggestion comes from Judy Townsend, who lives in Stratford-upon-Avon. Her grandmother, Ruth Farmer from South Africa, swears by nasturtiums:

Take two nasturtium leaves and one flower and eat them fresh to ward off colds. They are very peppery.

Anne McIntyre, the herbalist, would agree. In her book *The Complete Floral Healer* she says: 'Nasturtium has antimicrobial properties. It is particularly useful for chest infections, and because it also has decongestant properties it is well worth using to clear the phlegm that accompanies bronchial problems. The fresh juice or an infusion of the leaves relieves colds, catarrh and chronic bronchial congestion.'

The following two remedies were reported in the Women's Institute magazine *Home & Country*. They originally appeared in a section headed 'Recipes and Ancient Remedies' in *The Worcestershire Book*, produced by the Women's Institute:

Rosemary and cider

Boil a sprig of rosemary in half a pint [300 ml] of cider for fifteen minutes and drink it at bedtime as hot as possible. It is advisable to drink when in bed as it causes great perspiration.

Elderflower and peppermint

For colds, inflammations etc. take a handful of elderflower and one of peppermint, put in a jug and pour over it one and a half pints [900 ml] of boiling water. Let it steep for thirty minutes on the hob. Strain and sweeten with black treacle or honey. Drink hot in bed. The more you drink, the sooner the cure will be effected.

Mrs Grieve also gives the elderflower and peppermint remedy, specifying the use of dried elderflowers. She warns that heavy perspiration is likely to follow but insists that the patient will wake up well on the way to recovery and the 'cold or influenza will probably be banished within thirty-six hours'.

Elderflowers appear in another traditional English recipe in the form of a tea:

> *Take elderleaves or elderflowers and steep in boiling water. It helps catarrh, colds and inflammation.*

Christine Fletcher from Broughton in Hampshire used to watch her mother collect elderflowers and dry them on a tray in the sun. In winter they would take a few flowers, pour boiling water over them, add lemon and honey, and drink the mixture as a cold cure.

Not surprisingly, onions play their part in cold cures, and Christine still makes the onion sauce her grandmother used to give her as a child. She and her husband love the sauce and say that now, when they are both in their eighties, they rarely have colds.

> *She cooked three onions for two people, coarsely slicing them in a pan, adding a little water and a knob of butter. When the onions were soft, she added about a tablespoon of flour and a little milk, stirring until it thickened but remained a little runny.*

Here's another onion remedy from Anna Davies of London. It has also been recommended for treating coughs:

> *Dice an onion and sprinkle with sugar. Leave it overnight. In the morning, collect the syrup that has formed and pour it into a jar. Take one tablespoon of the syrup twice a day.*

A variation on this theme comes from Margaret Timms of Leamington Spa, who would cover the onion in honey rather than sugar.

Colds (chesty)

When she was a baby Marguerite Hughes from Birmingham had pneumonia, and one of her lungs 'closed'. As a result, she always had chesty colds during her childhood and found it hard to breathe at night. Her parents used to take a piece of thick rope out to the workmen laying a new road to soak in the tar. This would then be hung over Marguerite's bed to help her breathe. It's debatable whether or not sniffing tar is particularly good for you – perhaps if eucalyptus oil had been available it would have been better – but Marguerite not only survived, her lungs improved after she was about seven. Now in her eighties, with no recurring lung problems, she says she still enjoys a whiff of tar when there's some roadworks going on.

Sometimes, it was the grandfather rather than the grandmother who devised the cold cure. Pam Donaghue grew up in Liverpool in the 1950s, and her father, Samuel Thornley Horrocks, would make:

> *a cordial of fresh hot lemon squeezed into warm water, with a spoonful of treacle, another of honey and a tot of whisky.*

It had to be taken at bedtime and sipped slowly using a teaspoon. He would then rub camphor oil into the soles of his daughter's feet. 'Wonderfully warming,' remembers Pam. She used this remedy for her own children – and uses it still to this day.

Hot chicken soup, a favourite among the Jewish community, is a recurring remedy that is reputed to help with phlegm and has a disinfectant quality. Some say that it reduces the white blood cell count. It certainly is a sovereign remedy in all sorts of households all over

Europe. Ginger tea is another, but that has other uses too (*see also* Travel sickness and Vomiting).

Jennifer Clifton from Bristol recalls that when she was a child she would be given a bowl of very hot boiled onions, lavishly seasoned with salt and pepper and a knob of butter. A cloth would be placed over her head and the bowl, so it became a steam infusion. It was only when the onions had cooled that she was encouraged to eat them.

Other remedies were reported in the Women's Institute magazine *Home & Country* in August 1942, while the country was in the depths of the Second World War and struggling with wartime rationing. This remedy for a vinegar, cayenne and saltpetre rub appeared as an extract from *The Gleanings from Gloucestershire Housewives*:

Onion for colds.

> *Take half a pint [300 ml] of best vinegar, quarter oz [5 g] cayenne, half oz [15 g] saltpetre. Mix together in a bottle. Saturate a piece of flannel and rub on to the chest.*

It was followed by a remedy using cider and ground ginger:

> *Into a pint [600 ml] of hot draught cider stir a good teaspoonful of ground ginger.*

The remedy was followed by the instruction: 'Make a beeline (if you can) for bed.'

Colic in babies

Mrs Naina Ardeshani from Coventry has contributed a traditional Indian remedy for babies with colic:

> *Make a paste with the herb asafoetida and water and spread it around the baby's belly button.*

The Ayurvedic herb asafoetida (*Ferula assafoetida*), which is known paradoxically as both devil's dung and food of the gods, is renowned for treating the digestive system, especially bloating, cramps, flatulence and constipation from nervous indigestion. Sebastian Pole, an established Ayurvedic practitioner and herbalist, says: 'The skin is like the digestive system and absorbs much of what we put on it. Asafoetida is a warming anti-spasmodic, but it would be too hot internally for babies, hence this method which is a common one in India.'

In Britain gripe water – an infusion made from dill or fennel – is the traditional remedy. It is also common to lay an infant on your knee or over a warm hot water bottle and pat or rub their back.

If colic is a regular problem, breast-feeding mothers are usually asked to check their own diets.

Constipation

Everyone has their favourite solution for tackling constipation, but nowadays most people suggest that, in the first instance, you should drink double the amount of water you normally consume and make sure that you get plenty of exercise. Introducing bran or similar roughage into the diet is also common practice, although it is now known that if IBS (Irritable Bowel Syndrome) is suspected these insoluble fibres may be too harsh and could irritate the colon.

How different things were in 1842. Jean Gardyne from Sheepscombe in Gloucestershire found the two following remedies written by her great-great-grandmother, Eleanor Tristram, in the back of a cookery book dating from that time. The remedies were subsequently passed down through the family, and Jean offers these from notes her mother made:

THE BLACK DOSE
Senna leaves – 1½ oz [40 g]
Caraway seeds – 2 drachms
Bruised ginger – 3 drachms
Bruised cloves – 1 drachm

Add the ingredients to 1½ pints [900 ml] of water. Boil it until it becomes 1 pint [600 ml], strain it, add 12 oz [375 g] of Epsom Salts and 1 glass of gin. Dose: 2 drachms of mixture and the same of water.

OPENING MIXTURE
Take mint water – 3 oz [75 g] (steep mint leaves in hot water
  and strain)
Rhubarb powder and magnesia – each ½ drachm
Syrup of rhubarb – ½ oz [15 g]
Dose: 1 tablespoon to be taken first thing in the morning,
  repeat in 4 hours if it does not operate.

As Jean says: 'I think they both sound foul, and the black dose would have cleaned one out completely!' It must be mentioned that

Eleanor Tristram's fascinating cookbook also featured a recipe for orange brandy that starts: 'Take a gallon of best French brandy ...' This was obviously a very wealthy household.

Shirley Reynolds from the Isle of Wight suggests that liquorice offers a particularly attractive remedy for children with constipation:

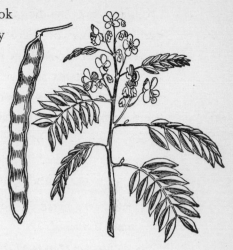

Senna for constipation.

> *Chop the liquorice into small pieces and place in a small glass bottle with hot water. Shake until the liquorice has started to melt.*

She benefited herself: 'It made a very good drink – and it certainly got things moving!'

Joan Griffiths from Huntingdon, Chester, subscribes to the liquorice remedy too. Her grandmother, Winifred Snelham, would buy liquorice powder from the chemist, add water to make a paste and dose her large family (seven sons and four daughters) every Friday night. Joan adds: 'How we all managed the after-effects of this with only one lavatory in the house, I don't remember.'

In Ireland, stoke, which is a kind of dark green-brown seaweed found attached to rocks only at low tide, was a traditional remedy for bowel regularity. It was boiled and strained and eaten as a vegetable. Robert McElhinney from Horn Head in County Donegal remembers it being served with potatoes. It was not only thought to aid regularity but also to contain iron.

Other recommendations included cabbage juice, figs (both fresh and in the form of the famous syrup of figs), curry, chilli, bitter chocolate and apples. Ripe juicy apples eaten at bedtime – or stewed apples taken at any time – have a laxative effect. Here is a compote recipe that combines several of these ingredients, taken from *A Kitchen Pharmacy* by Rose Elliot and Carlo de Paoli:

6 dried figs

6 prunes

1–2 eating apples

1 large pear (preferably Conference)

3 cloves (optional)

small piece of cinnamon stick (optional)

2 teaspoons apple juice concentrate or honey

Cover figs and prunes with water, soak for a few hours or overnight. Wash the apples and pear and cut, unpeeled, into thick slices, discarding the cores. Place in a saucepan with the figs, prunes, cloves and cinnamon and 10 fl oz [½ pint] of water. Bring to the boil and boil for 2–3 minutes. Then simmer over a low heat, without a lid, for 40–50 minutes or until the fruits are very tender and most of the water has evaporated, leaving a glossy syrup. Remove the cloves and cinnamon. Add honey or apple juice concentrate if necessary. Serve hot, warm or cold, perhaps with thick yoghurt.

Margaret Smith from Edinburgh recalls her mother giving her stewed and stoned prunes, made into a paste and mixed with a little senna powder. This is similar to a remedy that Jean Crossley of Marlborough also subscribes to: syrup of figs laced with senna. It is believed that senna has been cultivated in this country since about

1640, and its laxative properties are renowned. Another traditional remedy uses the pods on their own:

Take six dried senna pods and place in a small bowl of warm water. Leave them to soak overnight. Strain and sip the liquid.

A word of caution. Senna on its own can give griping pains and colic. It should not be taken when there is undiagnosed abdominal pain, and care should be taken about taking any laxative for a prolonged period.

An elderly aunt of mine used senna in a totally different way. Her husband was a sweet and charming man, but he did have a rather irritating, nervous little cough. It drove my aunt to distraction, and she was determined to cure it, although all the cough remedies she tried seemed to be ineffective. In desperation, she laced his tea with senna. Because of its highly laxative qualities, he simply did not dare to cough and within a few days the coughing habit was broken!

Consumption *see* Tuberculosis

Convalescence

From ancient times a period of convalescence was an accepted part of the recovery from most illnesses or injuries. Hippocrates, the father of medicine, advised it, so did Trotula and Hildegard of Bingen. Patients were encouraged to give their bodies time to recuperate properly. They were given nourishing foods, tonics and pick-me-ups, encouraged to undertake gentle exercise and were allowed plenty of rest and relaxation. The great Arabian physician

Avicenna, who followed Hippocrates, believed, as Hippocrates did, that hospitals should be beautiful environments in order to encourage healing, with clean air, fountains, flowers and music. Sadly, very few NHS hospitals live up to this ideal.

The tradition of convalescence continued until after the First World War, before pressure on time and budgets began to impinge. This may have proved to be a false economy, for if people are allowed to recover properly, they are less likely to suffer from ill health in the future.

Here is a pick-me-up for invalids found in Catherine Gould's great-great-grandmother's book of 'receipts', probably dating from 1860–70:

> *Take the yolk of a new laid egg, beat up well with ½ teaspoon of powdered sugar, 1 (teaspoon) of brandy, 1 wineglassful milk, 1 of water. Serve with sponge cake or plain biscuit.*

Possets were considered comfort foods for convalescents for many centuries. These were drinks of hot, sweetened milk curdled with wine – or with ale in poorer families – and spiced, perhaps with ginger. However, if a patient was convalescing from a fever or influenza the Victorians would probably have prescribed beef tea, which was also considered beneficial for anyone suffering from anaemia.

> *Trim any fat from half a pound [250 g] of good steak and cut into chunks. Pop it into a food processor and shred finely. Place the shredded steak in a bowl and add a good pinch of fresh or dried parsley, thyme, rosemary and marjoram. Add half a pint [300 ml] of water and cover with a pudding cloth. Place the bowl in a larger saucepan*

that you fill with water to the point where it reaches about halfway
up the outside of the bowl. Cover the saucepan with a lid. Bring the
water to the boil and then simmer for up to three hours. Check that
the saucepan doesn't dry out: top up with water whenever necessary.
When you remove the bowl and its pudding cloth, you can sieve
the mixture and skim off any fat. Allow to cool and serve. This can
be reheated.

Julia Campbell from Cupar in Scotland remembers being given beef tea when she was recuperating from heavy colds in her childhood in the 1920s and 1930s. She says that her mother would buy the best beef affordable at the time. The meat was boiled, then strained and salt was added. Her mother would also add a little Bovril to give more flavour.

And now for a small mystery: Margaret Smith from Edinburgh found a recipe for Egg Rum Emulsion, beautifully handwritten – although somewhat faded – on a small piece of paper in an old medicine chest. The chest is a family heirloom and at least a hundred years old. There's no way of knowing how old the remedy is, who wrote it or what it was for, but the consensus is, since it is not unlike an egg nog, that it was for building up a patient after illness.

Place 4 eggs in a basin without breaking them, pour over them the
strained Juice of 3 Lemons. Turn them in this for 3 days, on the 4th
day break up the shells and all and pour over this ½ pint [300 ml]
of Rum. Have in another basin ¼ lb [125 g] fine sugar (and) ½ pint
[300 ml] of Cream. Strain the eggs into this and bottle for use. Dose:
wineglass full three times Daily between meals.

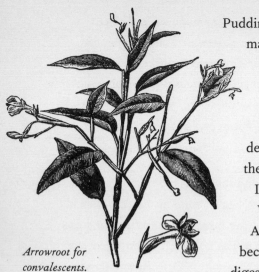

Arrowroot for convalescents.

Puddings, blancmanges and milky drinks made with arrowroot were also traditional foods for convalescents. Arrowroot (*Pueraria lobata*) was introduced into Britain in about 1730, and the name is thought to derive from the *aru-root* favoured by the Arnac Indians of South America. It comes predominantly from the West Indies, Central America, West Africa and the Far East. It was valued because it was nourishing and easily digestible, particularly in bowel complaints. Starch would be extracted from the lowest part of the stem – known as the rhizome – by pulping it with wooden mortars, and the milky extract was sieved and dried on clean sheets in the sun.

To make a drink, one tablespoon of arrowroot was made into a paste with a little cold milk or water, then carefully stirred while boiling milk was added. Lemon juice, sugar, wine or aromatics could be added. With plenty of milk, this would form a nourishing drink. If made thick, the mixture would cool and become a jelly.

As an aside, there are references in Mrs Grieve's *A Modern Herbal* to the mashed rhizomes of arrowroot being used as applications to wounds from poisoned arrows, scorpion and black spider bites. It seems unlikely, at first glance, that this knowledge would be useful to anyone in Britain, but it must be remembered that many Britons travelled across the globe from Tudor times onwards, and so it may have been a lifesaver.

Marjorie Melville, in service in Scotland in the second half of the nineteenth century, kept a recipe for a 'nourishing jelly for a sick person'.

> *Put into a stone jar or jug: a set of calves' feet cut in pieces; 1 quart [2 pints/1.2 litres] of milk; 5 pints [2.75 litres] of water; a little mace; half an ounce [15 g] of isinglass; a handful of hartshorn shavings.*

This ingredients list alone gives a fascinating insight into kitchens of the past. Isinglass comes from the swim bladders of fish and was widely used as a gelling agent before cheap production methods were found for gelatine, and hartshorn is a leavening agent, a precursor to baking soda and baking powder. The recipe continues:

> *Tie some brown paper over the jug and put into the oven. When done, strain and when cold remove fat. Some of it may be warmed with wine and sugar and it is good taken as broth with herbs.*

Marjorie followed this with a 'restorative':

> *1 oz [25 g] candied erring (sea holly) root*
> *1 oz [25 g] sage*
> *1 oz [25 g] pearl barley*
> *1 oz [25 g] rice*

> *Boil in 4 quarts [1 gallon/4.5 litres] of water till reduced by half. Take a dessertspoon with milk or wine.*

The Irish also harvested seaweeds to act as tonics, and they were reputed to be high in iron. Maureen Hanna from County Lough remembers carrageen moss, a kind of seaweed, being warmed in milk and then strained. It formed a thickened sauce that was used as a tonic. Robert McElhinney from Horn Head in County Donegal recalls that dulse, another type of seaweed, could be eaten straight from the seashore or after it had been laid out to dry.

Once patients were making progress and beginning to get back on their feet, it was common for a 'change of air' to be recommended. This would mean a stay in a different atmosphere. If you came from the city, then a period by the sea or in deep country would be called for. If you came from the country, you might opt for lakes or mountains and vice versa. Presumably this is where the old adage 'a change is as good as a rest' came from. No doubt the move would encourage deep breathing and, for someone who had been housebound for a time, act as a stimulant because they would meet new people and see new places.

Corns

I grew up knowing of a family remedy for corns, but sadly there's no trace of where it came from, although it possibly originated in South Wales. It uses liquorice to treat very hard skin on the feet:

> Grind three to four liquorice sticks and add in half a teaspoon of sesame oil or mustard oil. Smear the corn (or hard skin) with the resulting mixture before going to bed. Cover with socks. Use for several nights – or longer if necessary – until you can see the skin begin to soften and it is possible to lift the 'core' of the corn away.

Carola Augustin in Vienna suggested an alternative:

Take a slice of onion and leave it to soak in vinegar for a few hours. At bedtime place the onion over the corn and hold in place with a plaster, and leave overnight. Next morning, soak your foot in hot water. Repeat this remedy until the 'eye' of the corn comes away.

In her *Tried Favourites Cookery Book* (1948) Mrs E.W. Kirk gives the following remedy:

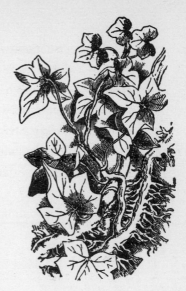

Ivy solution for corns.

Soak some young ivy leaves, say a dozen, in vinegar for three days, paint the solution on with a camel's-hair brush, then tie one of the leaves on the corn with thread. Change each night and morning, and in a few days the corn can be taken out without pain. After the corn has been taken out, continue the leaves for a day or two, in order to remove any little hardness that may remain.

Coughs

Even though printed cookery books have been available to buy for hundreds of years, many women in the past liked to make their own book of favourite recipes and remedies. Most have been thrown away, but some from Victorian times have survived, and one such, written by Lily Snow, has been kept by her granddaughter Betty

Smith from Sidmouth. Lily married twice, first to William Elliott of Brixton and later to Robert Pownall of Muswell Hill. There are several recipes for cough mixtures, but in some instances the quantities were measured not by weight but by cost, and so would be difficult to replicate today. Note too the use of laudanum, a derivative of opium, which was widely used in Britain and throughout Europe from the 1600s until late Victorian times.

LILY'S COUGH MIXTURE 1

2 pennyworth of the four following: laudanum, ether, nitre,
  peppermint
½ lb Flower's black treacle
½ pint vinegar

Warm treacle, add vinegar, stir well. When well mixed, add other ingredients and shake well. Dose for adult, 1 teaspoon night and morning. If very bad, a dose during the day. Half a teaspoon in water for a child.

LILY'S COUGH MIXTURE 2

1 pennyworth each of: laudanum, paregoric, oil of aniseed, oil
  of peppermint, ½ pint black treacle, 1 pint boiling water

In the Middle Ages the physicians of Myddfai offered a cough remedy based on agrimony (*Agrimonia eupatoria*):

Bruise agrimony in a mortar and mix the juice with boiling milk, strain and use.

Centuries later Nicholas Culpeper also suggested this usage, writing: 'This herb … helps the colic, cleanses the breast and rids away the cough.' Agrimony is still used by herbalists today, although more usually for strengthening the digestive system.

It is unsurprising that honey features in a lot of the old-fashioned remedies for coughs, because it is soothing, sweet and has antiseptic properties. More surprising is that so many remedies feature alcohol – or perhaps not in our chilly climate! Swedes also put in a couple of interesting appearances, along with good old onions. In the Devon WI cookbook, Mrs Spencer, from Marlborough, north Devon, suggests:

> *Skin some slices of swede. Put on a small plate, with a large plate underneath, and sprinkle with brown sugar. Leave for several hours with the upper plate tilted. The juice that drains off is soothing and palatable. Take a teaspoon when required.*

Agrimony for a cough.

Another recipe suggests cutting a hole in the middle of a swede and filling it with natural brown sugar. Leave it overnight so the juice collects, and sip it the following day.

The March 1932 issue of the WI magazine *Home & Country* includes this interesting remedy from France – and you can almost hear the accent – using honey and vinegar:

> *When the littles (or the bigs) cough, they often will not take things from the chemist. In a little hot water, make to cook two spoonfuls of honey and one (of) white fine vinegar. When it makes a very thick syrup, put in a bottle. Give him a spoon as a sweetie,*

or put it in a glass stirred with water as a cool drink, and the littles (and bigs) will say; 'Is there more?'

Here's another way to take honey:

Make a hole in a lemon and fill it with honey. Roast the lemon and then strain the juice. Take a teaspoon of the liquid frequently.

Herbalist Anne Stobart from Devon also suggests a honey remedy that is based on onions:

Peel and thinly slice one pound [500 g] of onions and half a pound [250 g] of garlic. Place in a dish and cover with a pint [600 ml] of sunflower oil. Cook slowly in the oven until the onion mixture is soft. Strain the mixture, add ¼ pint [150 ml] of honey and bottle the liquor. Stop the bottle firmly. Shake before taking the mixture.

If you run out of honey (which is not that unlikely if you use it as often as these traditional remedies suggest) you can always try this one from Carola Augustin:

Chop an onion very finely, put it on to a plate and cover with a generous sprinkling of sugar. Leave for an hour or two or even over night. A liquid develops. Pour it off into a glass and take a spoonful at regular intervals over the day. If the cough is severe, prepare a second batch during the day to take in the evening.

Carola gives this to her young daughter, Lisa, who reports that it is a bit sweet and strong but doesn't taste nasty. Her husband and son, however, prefer the following cough remedy:

Pour a pint [600 ml] of dark beer into a saucepan and bring to

*the boil. Remove from the heat and allow to cool a little. Add four
dessertspoons of honey to the warm beer. Drink it – but don't drive
afterwards!*

In some parts of Europe, especially in Germany, Austria
and Hungary, a cough jam is a well-known remedy:

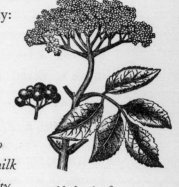

*Take a quantity of red elderberries and boil
them in a small amount of water. Simmer for
15 minutes and then strain through a fine sieve or
piece of muslin. Measure the resulting weight
and add the same amount of sugar (gelatine
sugar if you can find it or the usual kind). Put into
jars when cool. Take two teaspoons of the jam in milk
or tea or use as a spread. Elderberries have a quality
not dissimilar to aspirin.*

*Elderberries for
coughs.*

In Mrs Grieve's *A Modern Herbal* there are several recipes that
incorporate raspberries. Here is one for raspberry vinegar that she
quotes, taken from an old cookery book. We don't know just how
old the book was, but the language suggests it may be 100 or 150
years old.

*Put 1 lb [500 g] of fine fruit into a china-bowl, and pour upon it
1 quart [2 pints/1.2 litres] of the best white-wine vinegar. Next day,
strain the liquor on 1 lb [500 g] of fresh raspberries, and the following day do the same, but do not squeeze the fruit, only drain the
liquor as dry as you can from it.*

*The last time pass it through a canvas, previously wet with
vinegar, to prevent waste. Put it into a stone jar with 1 lb [500 g] of*

sugar to every pint [600 ml] of juice, broken into large lumps. Stir
it when melted, then put the jar into a saucepan of water or on a hot
hearth, let it simmer and skim it. When cold, bottle it.

The comment afterwards reads: 'This is one of the most useful preparations that can be kept in a house, not only as affording the most refreshing beverage but being of singular efficacy in complaints of the chest. A large spoonful or two in a tumbler of water. Be careful to use no glazed or metal vessels for it.'

Cracked heels

Not only are cracked heels unsightly, but they can also become painful if left untended. There are many remedies, but those that regularly come up use either sesame oil or ghee (clarified butter), either of which should be massaged into the heels at night. It would no doubt be a good idea to wear socks after applying the fat to protect your sheets.

Cuts (minor)

The belief that spiders' webs can help to heal cuts and wounds and to fight infections dates back thousands of years. Ancient Greeks applied spiders' webs to wounds, and there are further reports of their being used for wound dressings in the first century AD. There is evidence that spiders' webs were also used in the early seventeenth century: in Act 3, Scene 1 of *A Midsummer Night's Dream* (c.1596) Bottom, a rustic, is bewitched and given a donkey's head. In this

form he meets Titania, the queen of
the fairies, and her attendants, one
of whom is called Cobweb. 'I shall
desire you of more acquaintance,
good Master Cobweb. If I cut my
finger, I shall make bold with you,'
declares Bottom.

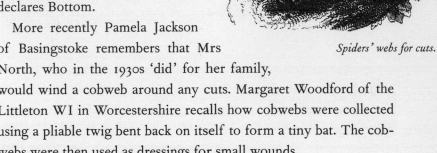

Spiders' webs for cuts.

More recently Pamela Jackson
of Basingstoke remembers that Mrs
North, who in the 1930s 'did' for her family,
would wind a cobweb around any cuts. Margaret Woodford of the
Littleton WI in Worcestershire recalls how cobwebs were collected
using a pliable twig bent back on itself to form a tiny bat. The cobwebs were then used as dressings for small wounds.

There haven't been many contemporary studies of the effectiveness of spiders' webs, but recent research has shown that spiders coat
their silk in antiseptic agents, and at Tufts University in Massachusetts
there are reports that researchers are looking at spiders' webs as
'scaffolds' for regenerating damaged knee ligaments.

Also from the Littleton WI, Mary Hilton suggested using the skin
of freshwater eels for dressings, although getting hold of one in the
first place may be difficult – and perhaps perilous – because the fish
are in such short supply these days.

Eileen Blenkinsop from Doncaster suffers badly from arthritis
and is in a wheelchair. Cuts and grazes are a constant hazard, and so
Eileen always carries a bottle of lavender oil in her handbag to treat
any minor accidents. She is such a fan of this remedy that she has
also put a bottle in the first aid box at her son's business premises.

Lavender's properties to both disinfect and stimulate tissue repair have been known and appreciated for thousands of years.

Here's a more unusual remedy from Mina Roberts of St Mawgan, Cornwall. She says: 'My mother, who is Hindu, taught me this and I use it myself and for my children.'

> *Take a handful of cotton wool and, somewhere safe, set light to it. Take the soot that is left and spread it on small cuts to cauterise them.*

Ayurvedic practitioner and herbalist Sebastian Pole says that the burned cotton remedy is well known and very ancient in India and that burned herbs are also used to stop bleeding, both internally and externally.

Cuts and wounds (serious or infected)

Sylvia Coppen-Gardner lives near the cathedral in Gloucester, and she recalls how her great-grandmother used to steep lily leaves in brandy and keep the bottle handy. She would use it to make a poultice for anything that required an antiseptic, such as infected cuts. Sylvia subsequently found the same remedy in a wonderful compendium called *The Family Magazine*, which came in two parts, the relevant one being 'The Body of Physick', dating from about 1741.

An alternative remedy is mentioned in Act 3, Scene 7 of *King Lear* (*c.*1605). The Earl of Gloucester has his eyes put out by the Duke of Cornwall, who has been spurred on to this torture by Regan, one of Lear's wicked daughters. Upon finding him distraught and bleeding, one of the servants says:

Go thou. I'll fetch some flax and whites of eggs
To apply to his bleeding face. Now, heaven help him!

Flax or linseed (*Linum usitatissimum*) is one of the oldest cultivated crops, grown for at least 7,000 years. Applied externally as a poultice, linseed is claimed to ease burns and boils, but I doubt if it would have proved particularly helpful in poor Gloucester's case.

Over the centuries field doctors have also used a number of surprising remedies for wounds, such as sphagnum moss, garlic, thyme and cabbage. Sphagnum moss (*Sphagnum cymbilifolium*) has a long history of being used as a dressing for wounds. According to Mrs Grieve's *A Modern Herbal* (1931), a Gaelic chronicle of 1041 relates that the wounded in the Battle of Clontarf 'stuffed their wounds with moss', and she quotes a report that Highlanders after the Battle of Flodden 'staunched their bleeding wounds by filling them with bog moss and soft grass'. The practice continued up to and including the Second World War, when so many medical materials were unavailable or in short supply. There are reports of women in the Land Army as well as members of the WI (see pages 205–9) collecting sphagnum moss from areas such as the Yorkshire Moors, the Lake District and the Wye Valley for use for dressing wounds. When there was a shortage of cotton wool, pads would be made of the absorbent moss, which was not only soft and comfortable but also had astringent and antiseptic qualities. The moss was cleaned and dried (preferably in the open air) and sometimes placed into muslin bags, sometimes sterilised

Crushed cabbage leaf poultices for wounds.

and, particularly in field hospitals, just made into compressed cakes. Garlic, reputed to be one of the best natural antiseptics, would sometimes be added.

Thyme – or rather camphor of thyme, also known as thymol – was used to medicate gauze and wool for surgical dressings because of its powerful antiseptic qualities. Cabbage was used too. Dr Valnet, who served in Indochina with the French army in the 1950s, often found himself short of essential medical supplies, and he resorted to the remedies used by the ancient physicians – Galen, Pliny and Hippocrates – when he was treating wounds that were gangrenous. He bound poultices of crushed cabbage leaves on to the wounds and reported that they would often heal without the need to resort to surgery or amputation.

As mentioned in the previous section on minor cuts, spiders' webs have been used for centuries for healing wounds, and in Hungary and Slovakia in the seventeenth century villagers in country areas would add the mould from bread – an unrefined form of penicillin – to the webs and place this over wounds.

There is also a tradition that raspberry leaves, which have astringent qualities, combined with the powdered bark of slippery elm (*Ulmus rubra*), which was much favoured by Native Americans, makes a good poultice for cleansing wounds, removing 'proud' flesh and promoting healing. This use of slippery elm is confirmed by *The Oxford Book of Health Foods*, which states: 'Extracts of slippery elm, being soothing and protective (demulcent and emollient) to surface body tissues ... externally [have] been employed for various skin conditions such as wounds, burns and boils.'

Dandruff

The cause of dandruff is still under debate. Some authorities suggest that the over- or under-production of oil by the sebaceous glands may be the reason; others believe that it is the result of an infection, and most cases seem to clear after the careful use of anti-fungal shampoos. In our grandmothers' time lavender or rosemary was often rubbed into the scalp, and a mixture of essential oils, such as cypress, juniper and cedarwood, are reputed to be useful.

Marjorie Melville, who was Anne Bisset's Scottish grandmother, wrote in her personal notebook that every trace of dandruff may be removed from the hair in a few weeks by using sulphur:

> *Take 1 oz [25 g] flowers of sulphur and add a quart [2 pints / 1.2 litres] of water — shake the liquid at intervals of two to three hours and every morning saturate the head with the clear liquid.*

She added another treatment:

> *wash the head once a week with a good tepid lather and rub into the scalp thereafter a little glycerine and borax.*

Just as fascinating are those remedies from the very distant past. In the Trotula Minor (see page 179), which possibly dates from the eleventh century, Trotula recommended this treatment against dandruff:

> *Take nettle seeds and soak them for two to three days in vinegar. Wash the hair, first with a good soap, then with this vinegar.*

She added a remedy for smoothing out thick hair:

> *Cook willow leaves, grind them, blend with olive oil and spread on
> your hair.*

The physicians of Myddfai recorded a medieval recipe for giving a
lift and golden tints to the hair:

> *Infuse bark of rhubarb in wine and wash your head therewith. Dry
> with a cloth, and then by the fire, or in the sun if it be warm. Do this
> again and often and the more beautiful will the hair become, and
> without injury to your hair.*

Depression

Severe depression – melancholy – was not understood or well treated in the past. Think of all those distressed souls in Victorian novels
who were locked away or compelled to 'haunt' the attics of larger
houses. However, for milder depressions – sadness and nervousness
– there were remedies, some of them very ancient.

For thousands of years in India and throughout the Middle East
the oils of roses and of jasmine, both costly and used in perfumery,
have been prized for their medical properties, including as anti-
depressants. These mood enhancers were used in vaporisers and
for massage. In Ayurvedic medicine jasmine is used for calming the
nerves and soothing emotional problems, while roses have a cooling
effect, calming the heart and lifting spirits.

In the West St John's wort (*Hypericum perforatum*) has been used
in traditional medicine for depression, anxiety, nervous tension and
insomnia for many centuries. According to *The Oxford Book of Health
Foods*, studies support many of the claims for this herb. However, it

may act adversely if it is taken alongside certain prescribed anti-depressants, and qualified advice should always be sought before combining traditional remedies and orthodox medicines.

Another herb long associated with dispelling sadness and boosting courage is borage (*Borago officinalis*). Pliny is reputed to have said that 'it maketh a man merry and joyful'. The Romans, and the Greeks before them, would use the flowers in a wine cup. Deborah Fowler, who created the Halzephron Herb Farm and shops in Cornwall, would recommend tincture of borage in cases of persistent depression, but in order to boost happiness she suggests infusing borage – and other herbs of choice – in Pimm's. Alternatively, she gives this remedy for a 'white wine cup':

75 ml [3 fl oz] sugar syrup
75 ml [3 fl oz] lemon juice
250 ml [9 fl oz] orange juice
4 tablespoons brandy
1 bottle semi-sweet white wine
3 long strips of cucumber peel
350 ml [12 fl oz] sparkling mineral water
3–4 stalks of borage, with flowers

Borage to boost courage.

Make sugar syrup by putting 75 g [3 oz] sugar in a small pan with 6 tablespoons of water. Bring slowly to the boil, then simmer gently, stirring, until the sugar has dissolved. Cool, then pour into a glass jug and add the fruit juices, brandy and wine. Add the cucumber peel and chill in the refrigerator for 2 to 3 hours. Shortly before serving, add the mineral water, plenty of ice and the borage.

In the Middle Ages the physicians of Myddfai believed that a wine cup would help soothe an irritable mind, as would celery:

If a man be irritable of mind, let him drink celery juice frequently; it will relieve his mood and produce joy.

Dermatitis

The twelfth-century mystic and healer Hildegard of Bingen offered this remedy for skin conditions in babies. It comes from Book 3, Chapter 28 of her *Physica*:

If any baby lying in its cradle is suffused and vexed with blood between the skin and the flesh so that it is greatly troubled, take new and recent leaves from the aspen [tree] and put them on a simple linen cloth and wrap the baby in the leaves and the cloth and put him down to sleep, wrapping him up so that he will sweat and extract virtue from the leaves; and he will get well.

Another remedy from the past is geranium (*Pelargonium*). These flowers came originally from the Cape in South Africa and arrived in England in the early seventeenth century at about the time of Charles I. Aromatherapists use the essential oil in the treatment of emotional disorders, depression and mood swings in particular, and for skin irritations, including eczema. It also acts as an insect repellent. Geranium is used in traditional French remedies, where it is turned into a lotion for skin eruptions:

Add 10 geranium leaves to one litre of boiling water. Simmer gently for one hour. Allow to cool and use as a poultice (that is, soaked into gauze and held in place with a light bandage). Do this

*four or five times a day. You can use camomile flowers in the same
way to soothe skin irritations.*

Another remedy found in several European countries is based on ice
and milk:

> *Crush ice cubes, place the mush in a glass and add milk. After
> a few minutes, place the mixture on to cotton gauze and apply to
> the afflicted area for at least three minutes. Change the compress,
> renewing the application every ten minutes.*

A further option is to follow the example of Gloria Jalil from
London. She keeps an aloe vera plant on her kitchen windowsill,
but apparently it never has a chance to grow very large because she
is always using its leaves. She breaks the leaf to access the 'gel' and
wipes it on any form of skin irritation. She also points out that it can
be used like shampoo because it will make hair very shiny.

See also Skin diseases.

Detoxification

Recently there has been a fashion for 'detoxing' or cleansing the
body of toxins. Many of the suggested regimes are mini-fasts or
light diets with just one or a couple of foods or juices consumed.
These can be helpful, but a more stringent, sudden or drastic fast
may be damaging, particularly if there is an existing health problem.
Newcomers to this kind of therapy should undertake any form of
fast only under the guidance of a fully qualified health practitioner,
such as a nutritionist or herbalist.

From the point of view of traditional medicine, what is interesting about the fashion for detoxing is how it echoes fasting therapy, which has been used throughout the world through the ages for healing. Noticing that sick animals instinctively go off their food, ancient peoples used fasting as a cure-all, and in earlier civilisations people would choose to fast not only during an illness but also on a regular basis in order to maintain good health, enhance concentration and mental powers and achieve longevity. In ancient Greece Hippocrates and Galen, who between them created the basis for modern medicine, both advocated regular fasts as part of a health regime.

Fasting not only rests the digestive system and those organs and glands involved in the digestive process, but it is also thought to cleanse the blood. After the first twenty-four hours the toxins and other waste matter that have accumulated in the intestines and bloodstream start to be eliminated, and as the waste is off-loaded, the blood assumes its correct acid/alkaline balance. The optimum time for a fast suggested in the Indian Ayurvedic tradition and in traditional Chinese medicine is seven days, which is believed to be the length of time that it takes to clear the bloodstream and the lymph systems of their waste.

In *The Tao of Health, Sex and Longevity* Daniel P. Reid quotes the tenth-century Sung Dynasty physician Chang Tsung-cheng, who recommended cleansing the colon with fasting for a range of ailments, including indigestion and constipation, breathing problems, headaches and fevers, stiff and painful joints and – interestingly – mental and emotional abnormalities. He wrote: 'All physicians know that the unobstructed circulation of fresh blood and vital energy are the most important factors in health. But if the stomach and bowels are blocked, then blood and energy stagnate.'

Perhaps more enjoyable than fasting is to undergo a sweating regime. The Finns are renowned for introducing the sauna to the world, but the tradition of steaming the body for cleansing, detoxifying and relaxation is far more widespread and has a long pedigree. Native Americans from many different tribes built sweat lodges. These would be either oblong or dome shaped and were usually built from tree branches on bare earth and covered with clay, blankets or skins to keep in the heat. Hot stones were placed in a shallow pit inside the lodge, which would be completely dark. A fire-keeper would pour water on the stones to increase the steam.

The sweat lodge was known in Mexico and Guatemala too, where it was called a *temazcal*. The tradition predates the Spanish conquest, and the lodges were used for therapeutic cleansing. Often herbs were thrown on to the stones to give a fragrant and beneficial steam vapour. The *temazcal* remains popular but now more as a bathing facility, using soap and mainly in the evenings when cooler air provides a counterbalance. Wet steam baths were – and are – to be found in other cultures, including the famous Turkish bath, the *hammam*, the Russian *banya*, the Jewish *shvitz* and, in Africa, the *sifutu*. Turkish steam baths were popular in Britain too, and are still to be found, although mainly in the older gyms and gentlemen's clubs.

In Japan and the Far East bathhouses have always been popular as social meeting places as well as places for cleansing and relaxation. Most Japanese now have baths in their homes, but in the past whole families would attend the public baths together. The body was cleansed scrupulously before entering the bath to wallow in warm water. Nowadays, public bathhouses also offer Jacuzzis, steam rooms and saunas.

The origins of the Finnish sauna are ancient, perhaps as early as the fifth century. The sauna was a sacred place and, since it gave a sterile as well as a warm, comforting environment, it was where women retired to give birth, a practice that continued until quite recent times. Gradually the sauna became an integral part of Finnish life, a place to relax physically and mentally. Even now, most Finns take a sauna at least once a week, and saunas are to be found not only in private homes but also in business premises, in recreational locations, such as by lakes and forests, and even at the country's parliament building

A typical sauna is a wooden room with a special stove containing the hot stones that will produce the steam, taking the temperature, usually 70–78°C (158–172°F), up to a maximum of about 100°C (212°F). Water is sprinkled on to the stones to enhance the steam, making the sauna hotter. Clothing of any type, including swimwear, or even towels is rarely worn. Bunches of twigs – traditionally, silver birch – may be used to gently beat the body, helping to relax the muscles. At the point when the heat becomes overwhelming, sauna users will jump into a plunge pool, a lake or even roll in the snow. After cooling down and perhaps taking a drink, it is usual to return to the sauna for another or even several more sessions.

Saunas have some health benefits. The dry heat has been shown to prevent the common cold and to help asthma and bronchitis sufferers. It also improves microcirculation and helps rheumatism. As a relaxing therapy it has been shown to reduce high blood pressure, but care must be taken because the shock of moving from one extreme of temperature to another can be quite severe. It may

also be dangerous for people with angina and anyone
with a heart condition.

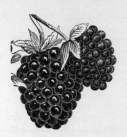

Diarrhoea

There are dozens of remedies relating to diarrhoea,
some more effective than others, and there is a consensus that sweet things, including chocolate, exacerbate
the condition.

*Blackberries for
diarrhoea.*

Blackberries, which can still be found in many hedgerows, provide a remedy for dysentery and diarrhoea. Obviously, they can be
eaten straight from the bramble but here is a delicious cordial:

> *To make a blackberry cordial: press the fruit from ripe black-
> berries. Add 2 lb [1 kg] sugar to every quart [2 pints/1.2 litres] of
> the resultant juice. You can also add a pinch of nutmeg or cloves.
> Boil all the ingredients together for a short time. Allow to cool.
> Add a little brandy.*

Dr Henry Oakeley, a Fellow of the Royal College of Physicians,
who has taken a particular interest in herbal medicine, adds: 'The
bark of the [blackberry] root and the leaves contain much tannin and
may have long been used as an astringent and tonic, proving a valuable remedy for dysentery and diarrhoea.'

Blackberries are often paired with apples, which are known to
alleviate constipation. Perhaps when there is no existing condition
of either diarrhoea or constipation, the two are paired together to
balance each other out.

Other remedies that have been suggested for diarrhoea include two to three cups of tea made from raspberry leaves, black tea with no sugar or milk, a purée of bananas (made by mashing them) to which a few drops of lemon have been added, a glass of fresh orange juice mixed with a teaspoon of salt, or a glass of cola mixed – again – with salt and whisked to remove any bubbles.

An unusual remedy comes from the *Tried Favourites Cookery Book* by Mrs E.W. Kirk, published in 1948:

A tablespoon of raw arrowroot, mixed with a little sifted sugar and sufficient cold milk to just swallow easily.

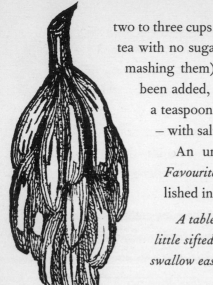

Bananas for diarrhoea.

She adds: 'Diarrhoea of many weeks' standing has been cured by this.' For more about arrowroot see the main article on Convalescence.

Dysentery was a feared condition, endemic in the trenches during both the Crimea War and the First World War. Mrs Kirk recommended the following treatment:

1 egg, 1 teaspoon sugar. Beat the egg and sugar very lightly and swallow in one gulp if possible. It soothes the inflammation in the stomach and intestines, and forms a transient coating to these organs until gradually the disease is removed. 2, or even 3, eggs a day may be used in this way, and the patient kept very quiet, with very light diet other than the egg.

Mary Whittington who, with her family, ran a luxurious hotel on the Cornish cliffs, would treat any guest with diarrhoea with a hot water drink, laced with sugar and salt. The combination of sugar and salt stimulates fluid absorption from the small intestine and counteracts the secretion caused by the 'bugs'. The following simple remedy of sugar and salt was hailed by the prestigious medical journal *The Lancet* as one of the greatest medical breakthroughs of the twentieth century. It has saved countless lives worldwide in conditions where diarrhoea could have proved fatal: 'Take one litre [1¾ pints] of water, one teaspoon of salt and eight teaspoons of sugar.'

Dog bites

Thankfully, in these days of strict animal quarantine, the possibility of being bitten by a rabid dog is extremely remote. However, this was not always the case in Britain, and this remedy, printed in the *Scots Magazine* of 1739 and sent to me by David Orr of Kirriemuir, Angus, shows how people would have dealt with such a bite.

> *Take twenty-four grains of Native Cinnabar, twenty-four grains of Factitious Cinnabar, and sixteen grains of the finest Musk; reduce each of these, separately, to an exceeding fine powder; then mix them well together in a glass of rum, arrack, or brandy, and drink it off, all at one dose, as soon as possibly you can after you are bit; and take a second dose thirty days after the first.*
>
> *But suppose you should happen to be bit by a dog, and should neglect taking any remedy soon after the bite, upon a supposition that the dog was not mad; in such a case, as soon as any symptoms of madness appear in the person, by that neglect, they must take a dose as soon as possibly they can after those symptoms appear; and instead*

of taking a second dose thirty days after the first, as in the other case mentioned above, the second dose must be given three hours after the first, which, by throwing the patient into a profound sleep and strong perspiration, will thoroughly cure the bite of any mad animal, though the distemper were in the very last stage.

According to the editors of the magazine, this remedy had 'not failed in the cure of any one person, out of many, who have taken it'.

Earache

A researcher into the life of Julian of Norwich, the woman mystic and spiritual authority who lived from 1342 to 1416, discovered an ancient remedy for earache. In a thirteenth-century English herbal, she found a recommendation to:

> dip a clove of garlic in honey and to insert it into the ear every night for a week.

Interestingly, garlic also appears in a number of recipes for food during the period. Things have moved on since the thirteenth century, however, and nowadays this remedy would not be recommended. It's very important not to put into the ear either hard substances or sticky mixtures that will dry. One country GP had a number of cases where he had to extract cloves of garlic that had become lodged in the ear canal after patients had pushed them in too far. Garlic, like peas and beans, will swell in liquid and start to grow. It may be an antiseptic, but in this sort of use it is more like to cause an infection than otherwise.

Mina Roberts from St Mawgan, Cornwall, has a solution that still offers all the healing properties of garlic without the hazard of growth.

> Fry garlic gently in a little oil. When it has cooled – become warm rather than very hot – dip a ball of cotton wool into it. Place the cotton wool ball gently into the affected ear and leave overnight.

Onion is the same genus as garlic, *Allium*, and provides an alternative remedy:

Slice an onion and then press each slice with the flat side of the knife to extract the onion's liquid. Gather both the onion pulp and the liquid and wrap it in a small cotton cloth (or handkerchief) and hold to the ear for 30 minutes or more. Your ear may improve, although your arm will then be tired!

Carola Augustin suggested the above, and she also swears by parsley:

Take a handful of parsley, chop it and squeeze it. Put the pulp on to a piece of gauze, wrap it to make a pad and place on the ear. Parsley is both anti-inflammatory and antiseptic.

Lavender offers a more gentle solution:

Warm a teaspoon of olive oil. Add two drops of the essential oil of lavender. Soak a plug of cotton wool in the mixture and place gently into the ear.

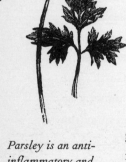

Parsley is an anti-inflammatory and antiseptic.

Many older people also remember their mothers or grandmothers filling a sock with household salt, placing it in the oven until warm and then placing it against the affected ear.

Eyes (tired and sore)

Wild plants are rarely considered to be in the same league as specially cultivated herbs, and yet some have very specific medicinal properties. A perfect example is ground ivy (*Glechoma hederacea*), which can be found in hedgerows, woodland copses and on wet, rough pasture. The plant has a strong aroma and would sometimes be added to hops in home-made beer to give it a bitter tang. But according to Peter Cooper, who for many years produced the nature notes for parish magazines in Cornwall, a more important use was in a lotion to soothe sore eyes. He wrote:

> *Gamekeepers whose eyes became inflamed by exposure to gunpowder fumes discovered that they could obtain relief by using an infusion of ground ivy made with boiling water to bathe them. The notion is believed to have originated from itinerant gypsies.*

Peter explained that juice expressed from the plant was also applied to bruises and black eyes and made into a poultice to help heal abscesses and tumours.

Cool or tepid tea has traditionally been used to relieve eye strain. The tea can be strained from the teapot and soaked into pads, which are applied to the eyes, or cool, used teabags can be gently squeezed out and applied directly to the eyes. Either way, put your feet up and relax with the tea pads in place for half an hour.

My own family's remedy to remove something in the eye – a stray eyelash or a bit of grit – was to chop a very large fresh onion. As your eyes water, the foreign body should float away. I can vouch for the effectiveness of this method. To soothe the eyes after the foreign body had been removed, a weak tea made from elderflowers and allowed to cool thoroughly, was a well-known remedy in parts of the Midlands and possibly elsewhere.

Ground ivy for sore eyes.

Fainting

During the Victorian period fashion decreed that well-dressed women should wear very tight corsets, which were laced to a point where women's waists were minute but their breathing was constricted and shallow, and any high emotion caused a fluttering heart and, all too frequently, fainting. Rather than opting for more comfortable styles of dress, Victorian women would keep a handy supply of smelling salts. These salts were usually a compound of ammonium carbonate because the ammonia would agitate the mucous membrane that lines the nose and throat, triggering deep inhalations that would revive the patient. Alternative names for smelling salts were sal volatile and the spirit or salts of hartshorn, the name originating in the days when the main source of ammonia was the antlers of male deer (or hart).

An onion makes a more natural 'smelling salt' and this was used in country areas:

> Chop the onion and persuade the patient to inhale it until tears come.

The ammonia in the onion dilates the blood vessels, thereby increasing the blood supply to the brain.

The advice for coping with someone who has fainted has changed slightly over the years. Nowadays we try to put the person's head between their knees to allow blood to flow back towards the brain, but in earlier times it was recommended that the patient be kept lying down with the head flat and feet raised. According to a little booklet that was produced by Sunlight Soap – which was popular in the first half of the twentieth century – the patient's face should then be flicked with a wet towel and smelling salts applied to the nostrils. As soon as the patient recovered sufficiently to swallow, a warm drink was suggested – ah, the power of the cup of strong tea.

Feet (tired and sore)

Ninety-four-year-old Mrs H. from Bakewell, Derbyshire, is a great exponent of the value of the herb comfrey (*Symphytum officinale*) and keeps some in her garden so that she can use it regularly. Her remedy for sore feet is to soak the broad comfrey leaves in a large bowl of hot water into which she then puts her feet.

Comfrey is also known as knitbone, and it has been used in herbal medicine for centuries – there is even a record of its use in the first century. Internally, it was used for bronchial disease, gastric ulcers, irritable bowels and rheumatism. It has been applied externally to broken bones (hence its name), bruises and sprains. Recent studies have found that comfrey contains allantoin, which is associated with tissue healing, and it is still used in ointments for sprains and bruising in Germany.

A much more modern remedy for tired feet is to use vodka. Lindsay Gill of Jersey insists that if you have been on your feet all day and they are becoming sore, you should rub them with a little vodka, which will numb them. Apparently, top models do this, too.

A thyme footbath is a traditional French favourite because of the herb's antiseptic properties:

Add two teaspoons of dried or fresh thyme to half a litre [17 fl oz] of water. *Simmer for 10 minutes, allow to cool and then soak the feet for half an hour.*

After a long walk you can make a footbath for your tired feet from walnuts.

Add a handful of ground nuts to half a litre of water [17 fl oz], simmer for quarter of an hour. Strain and allow the water to cool and add a handful of salt. Soak your feet for 10 minutes, then massage them with lemon juice to soften any inflamed skin.

Thyme for sore feet.

Fevers

The widely known remedy for both adults and children with a light fever is sponging down, sometimes with a drop or two of vinegar added to the water. If the fever was more severe, more extreme measures would have been employed. Anna Davies from southeast London tells of a dramatic remedy for the raging temperature that accompanies typhus or pneumonia, often with the loss of voice. It is not unlike using a compress (see page 229). She recounts:

Wet a bed sheet with cold water and wrap the patient up completely, including the head. Just leave an opening for the mouth and nose. Cover the patient with lots of blankets and let the patient lie in this cocoon until they feel hot again.

Anna says that this remedy was used successfully by her grandmother,

Waleria Kwasna, who was a teacher in the late 1920s in northeast Poland, now part of Lithuania. She became very ill, was running a high temperature and lost her voice completely. People feared for her life as there were no antibiotics at that time, and the illness persisted. After the wet sheet cure she regained her voice immediately and the fever left her completely.

A similar remedy is suggested by David Orr from Kirriemuir in Angus. In a volume called *The Scotsman's Library* (1825) he discovered a cold cure that is, in fact, designed to help a fever.

> *John Campbell Forrester, of Harries [Isle of Harris] makes use of this singular remedy for a cold. He walks into the sea up to the middle, with his clothes on, and immediately afterwards goes to bed in his wet clothes, and then laying the bed clothes over him, procures a sweat, which removes the distemper; and this, he told me, is his only remedy for all manner of colds.*

A remedy for fever that uses cold water and vinegar compresses is popular in Germany, Austria and parts of Italy, and it is used especially for treating the high temperatures that children tend to get when they have, for example, measles or flu. The advantage is that, unlike any drug remedy, this has no side effects at all. However, if there are more worrying signs or symptoms, such as neck pain and an aversion to bright lights, a doctor must be consulted quickly. Carola Augustin in Vienna and her sister-in-law Marina, who is Italian, both suggested the following treatment:

> *In a shallow bowl, add 5 dessertspoons of vinegar to a litre [1¾ pints] of cold water. Take linen strips (or tea towels or wide bandages), dunk them in the water and squeeze them out gently.*

Place the strips around the lower legs of the patient, that is, between the knee and ankle. Wrap dry towels around the compresses and cover the patient with a warm duvet. Allow them to relax for half an hour. Then check to see if the compresses have dried. If so, repeat the exercise until the temperature has reduced. It is easy for a patient to become dehydrated when they have a high fever, so it is also important to ensure that the patient is drinking plenty of fluids – water or teas – to help sweat the fever out of the system.

In her book *Folk Medicine* Frances Kennett suggests that on the English/Welsh borders pearl barley was used for lesser fevers:

Take two ounces [50 g] of pearl barley and five pints [2.75 litres] of water. Wash the barley in the water, then set the water aside. Boil the barley in half a pint [300 ml] of fresh water for five minutes. Add the set-aside water and boil again until it reduces to two pints [1.2 litres]. Strain off the liquid and drink it to reduce fevers and inflammations.

A quicker remedy, according to Carola Augustin, is parsley tea:

Take a bunch of parsley and chop it, leaves and stems together. Use one dessertspoon of the chopped parsley to one large cup of water. Put into a saucepan and bring to the boil. Simmer for two to three minutes, strain and drink.

Apple water is an old English remedy, and a recipe appears in Mrs Grieve's *A Modern Herbal* that suggests thinly slicing three or four apples without peeling them, then boiling them in a saucepan with a quart (2 pints/1.2 litres) of water and a little sugar until the slices become soft. The apple water will then require straining and it can be taken cold.

If the fever is intermittent the medieval physicians of Myddfai suggested this remedy:

> *Take dandelion and fumitory infused in water, first thing in the morning. Then about noon take wormwood in tepid water, at ten draughts. Eat wheaten bread, oatcakes and young chickens but no milk foods. If the fever does not end, put the patient in a bath when the fever is on him, and give him an emetic, which will then act more strongly.*

Flatulence

There is a general consensus that some high fibre foods – lentils, leeks, peas, beans and bran, for instance – can create excessive wind and bloating. A traditional Irish folk remedy for 'wind in the stomach', described by Frances Kennett in *Folk Medicine*, consists of half a pint (300 ml) of milk (probably warmed) with four teaspoons of soot. This sounds unlikely but, as she points out, carbon is sometimes prescribed for flatulent conditions of the stomach and intestines.

Another remedy comes from Kae Chapman-Turner:

> *Put two teaspoons of caraway seeds in a cup or mug, add hot water to make a tea. Allow to steep for a couple of minutes, strain and sip.*

The seeds of fennel (*Foeniculum vulgare*) have long been regarded as a carminative for 'wind'. In India the seeds are toasted and then chewed after a meal to help digestion. In Britain a tea is made from the seeds to treat everything from hiccups to colic. Scientific research bears out the anti-spasmodic properties of fennel seeds and has shown that they also contain potassium, carotenes, vitamins E and B complex and a small amount of vitamin C.

Fennel was one of the nine sacred herbs recognised by Anglo-Saxon herbalists, and its range of powers was lauded in this verse from *The Englishman's Doctor* (1608):

In Fennel-seed, this vertue you shall find,
Foorth of your lower parts to drive the winde,
Of Fennel virtues foure they do recite,
First it hath power some poysins to expell,
Next, burning Agues will it put to flight,
The stomack it doth cleanse, and comfort well:
And fourthly, it doth keepe, and cleanse the sight,
And thus the seede and herbe doth both excel.

Fennel seeds are a carminative.

See also Indigestion.

Fungal infections *see* Toenails

Gastroenteritis in babies

Angela Moules from Salisbury is now a ninety-year-old grand-mother. She recalls her training as a nurse at Great Ormond Street Hospital for Sick Children in the 1930s when they would give babies suffering from gastroenteritis a weak solution of tea along with pulped and sieved grated apple. The tannin in the tea was supposed to line their stomachs, she explains. To toddlers they would give tea-spoons of grated raw apple, skins included – Granny Smith apples were the preferred variety – because the pulp would fill their stom-achs so they could neither vomit nor pass loose stools.

In the Philippines an age-old remedy was to give babies or small children the water in which the daily rice had been boiled. Gloria Jalil from London says that when the rice was boiled for long enough the liquid became like a milk, which was not only easy to digest but helped settle the child's stomach.

A more traditional country remedy for relieving infant diarrhoea and one that is found all over Europe is a purée of cooked carrots, made by scraping a pound (500 g) of carrots and boiling them until they are soft in 1½ pints (900 ml) of water, then blending. The quan-tity of water will have reduced as the carrots boiled, so the next step is to top up the water to make 1½ pints (900 ml) again. Allow the mixture to cool before putting it into a bottle to feed the sick child.

Gout

There are lots of Victorian cartoons of rich old gentlemen with bandaged big toes, supposedly suffering from gout, a disease that was believed to be the result of too much good food and brandy. Although the big toe is the joint most frequently affected by this particularly painful form of rheumatic disease, gout can, in fact, afflict any joint, and it often takes the form of 'attacks', difficult to predict, which last for anything from three to ten days. Surprisingly, it is still quite common and affects one in 200 people, predominantly men. It is actually caused by the build-up of uric acid in the bloodstream, and it is unusual among women, who tend to have lower levels of uric acid in their blood.

The remedies for gout tend to be similar to those for rheumatoid arthritis. Celery seeds, garlic and artichokes are often recommended, as are turnips and leeks, both of which are credited with eliminating uric acid.

According to Michael van Straten and Barbara Griggs in their book *Superfoods*, the Swedish botanist Linnaeus (1707–78) recommended strawberries, claiming that he had personal experience of their efficacy, curing himself from gout by eating a diet composed almost entirely of strawberries. Cherries also have a special affinity to gout, because they have a long-held reputation for removing toxins and cleaning the kidneys. In their book *Kitchen Pharmacy* Rose Elliot and Carlo de Paoli point out that it is their cleansing properties that make cherries

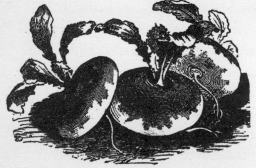

Turnips can help eliminate uric acid.

particularly valuable in the treatment of gout, adding that in ancient times, in both the East and West, cherries were believed to rejuvenate the body.

See also Rheumatism (rheumatoid arthritis).

Grazes

Pamela Jackson from Basingstoke had her childhood scratches and grazes treated with the mouldy paper from the top of a jar of jam. As she says, the mould was a primitive form of penicillin, and this possibly explains why other people have memories of using the mouldy cloth in which cheese had been wrapped. These remedies have an extraordinarily long pedigree. The earliest recorded use of antibiotics was by Egyptian physicians who used mouldy bread to treat wounds in about 2700 BC.

More recently, Elnora Fingland, a former nurse who lived in Birmingham in the 1950s and 1960s, resorted to iodine:

> *Dilute one teaspoon of iodine, which is a strong antiseptic, to one pint [600 ml] of water and wash the affected area.*

I remember this remedy from personal experience, because 'Fing', as I and some of her former charges used to call her, would sometimes look after me when my parents were working. On these occasions, I would be very careful not to bruise or graze myself because the iodine would sting like anything, and my eyes water at the very memory of it. Although it has great disinfectant properties and was effective, it is little wonder that it went out of fashion.

See also Cuts and wounds (serious or infected).

Haemorrhoids

A traditional remedy in France employs chestnuts to treat haemorrhoids. Chestnut trees (*Castanea*) were introduced into France from India in the fourteenth century, and there are records of chestnuts being used for circulatory problems from the fifteenth century onwards. The trees' anti-inflammatory properties were identified, and the chestnuts, leaves and flowers were all made into capsules. Here is the recipe for a chestnut cream:

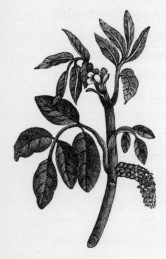

Walnut leaves for haemorrhoids.

Add one to two teaspoons of ground chestnuts – either fresh or dried – to a cup of boiling water. Allow it to infuse for ten to fifteen minutes. When cool enough, apply the cream to the haemorrhoids.

In *Kitchen Pharmacy* Rose Elliot and Carlo de Paoli maintain that tea made from walnut (*Juglans*) leaves will provide an enema that can be used for haemorrhoids or piles:

Make a tea using 2 teaspoons of walnut leaves to 1 pint [600 ml] of water. Use as an enema, holding the water as long as comfortable before discharging it.

Mrs Hewitt in the Devon WI cookery book points out that distilled witch hazel is astringent and can be dabbed on to reduce swellings and ease haemorrhoids. Certainly witch hazel (*Hamamelis*) has not only astringent but also antiseptic properties.

Another recommendation is to take a nettle tea:

Gather the tender tops of stinging nettles. Cover with water and boil for about 15–20 minutes. Strain and drink the liquid. A small amount of sugar may be added.

Halitosis

There are two major causes of halitosis or bad breath: poor dental hygiene or a digestive disorder. Smoking is another culprit – but we all know the remedy for that.

Dental hygiene is mentioned under Teeth cleaning (see page 148), but there are a number of other ways of freshening the mouth. Rinsing the mouth with warm water to which half a lemon has been added is refreshing. Chewing a few leaves of peppermint (*Mentha piperita*) will freshen both the mouth and breath. An effective mouthwash, which you can also use as a gargle, can be made by adding 30 drops of a tincture of myrrh to a glass of warm water.

Eating certain foods, such as garlic and strong spices, will give your breath a strong odour, which can be offset by chewing fresh parsley. Other useful herbs include coriander, sweet basil, rosemary, thyme, cloves, fennel and aniseed.

If your halitosis persists it may well be caused by a digestive disorder, in which case it will need further investigation and possibly a visit to a doctor.

See also Constipation; Indigestion; Teeth cleaning.

Hangover (and related stomach upsets)

Cornwall is famous not only for its surf beaches, Arthurian legends and pasties, but also for its china clay. China clay – or kaolin – was discovered in mid-Cornwall in 1746 by a Quaker apothecary called William Cookworthy (1705–80). He subsequently set up a pottery to produce porcelain, previously made only in China. Soon a number of pits opened to supply other renowned potteries, including that of Josiah Wedgwood.

Then, as now, china clay was mined in open-cast pits, where the clay would be washed out from the granite substructure using high-pressure water hoses. Soon other uses were found for china clay, notably for filling and coating paper. If one of the men who worked in the pits had a hangover or an upset stomach from overindulgence, he would scoop up some of the slurry from the clay stream and drink it. Nowadays, china clay is also used by the pharmaceutical industry. It forms the common base powder to which active ingredients are added for all kinds of pills and potions.

It has also been recorded that the Arnhem Land Aborigines in Australia would – and still do – eat small balls of white clay with pieces of earth from termite moulds to treat diarrhoea and stomach upsets. Apparently, the clay and the termite earth have similar properties to kaolin. And until quite recently, a mixture of kaolin and morphine was a regular treatment for upset stomachs, and bottles were available from pharmacists without prescription.

If anyone is looking forward to a party or expecting a bout of heavy drinking, herbalists still recommend milk thistle (*Silybum marianum*), which is a restorative for the liver. The idea is to take milk thistle tablets before you go out, and take them again should you over-indulge. Milk thistle also helps the bad breath associated with a hangover.

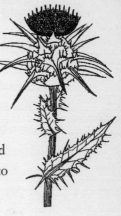

If the worst has happened and you have a hangover the traditional remedy is 'hair of the dog'. Scientifically – or even in terms of plain common sense – this is not a good idea. If your system is already overloaded with alcohol, pouring in still more will only delay the inevitable and uncomfortable detoxing. At some stage your liver is going to respond to the abuse.

An alternative – and there are many – is olive oil and a raw egg:

Milk thistle is a restorative for the liver.

> *Take a raw egg and a slug of olive oil and mix them into a glass of milk. No matter how disgusting this looks, you are meant to drink it.*

An unusual herbal cure is borage (*Borago officinalis*), usually considered both an aphrodisiac and an anti-depressive. However, Richard Mabey, author of *Food for Free*, avers: 'I can testify to one case, at least, where the dried leaves proved of inestimable value as a hangover cure, first used as an inhalant in hot water and then, in desperation, drunk. It really did seem to have a remarkably exhilarating and head-clearing effect.'

Hayfever

Many of the symptoms of this disorder may be alleviated by the remedies shown under Colds (see page 37). However, there is a persistent belief that hayfever can be avoided by taking a tablespoon of locally produced honey every day for the three months prior to the pollen season. This was suggested by, among others, June Richardson of Glasgow, although she has no experience of its success.

Headache

There are many reasons why someone develops a headache: anxiety, stress, muscular tension in the neck and shoulders, constipation, overindulgence, allergies and insomnia. Where possible, it is often useful to identify the cause.

The twelfth-century mystic and healer Hildegard of Bingen differentiates between different kinds of headache and suggests appropriate remedies. For a headache 'arising from melancholia' she recommends a mixture containing mallow (*Malva*), sage (*Salvia*) and olive oil; failing that, vinegar used as a compress on the head. Migraine, however, requires more exotic ingredients such as aloe, myrrh and poppy oil mixed with flour. Sabina Flanagan, who wrote an authoritative biography of Hildegard, suggests that the qualities of the plants – the heat of aloe, dryness of myrrh, coldness of poppy and blandness of the flour – would combine to allay the headache. It is believed that Hildegard herself suffered from migraine, and some authorities suggest that her visions were linked to the 'migrainous experiences' that she endured.

More recently, Mary Ramm, a member of Littleton WI in Worcester suggested:

collect leaves from the feverfew plant, pour on boiling water and allow them to steep to make a tea to help with a headache.

The Oxford Book of Health Foods by J.G. Vaughan and P.A. Judd reports that feverfew (*Tanacetum parthenium*) has a long history as a medicinal herb. It has been used to induce menstruation and aid placenta expulsion since Roman times, and it has many other uses, not least, as its name suggests, to lower temperature. The authors also point out that the active chemical constituents in the leaf (and stem) appear to inhibit the hormone seratonin, which is thought to trigger migraine, and they add: 'There is considerable clinical and experimental evidence to support its use as an anti-migraine agent, although it should not be taken for more than four months without medical advice.'

Lavender applied to the temples for headaches.

Lavender applied to the temples or in a cold compress applied to the forehead or the back of the neck were remedies used in Victorian times, and probably earlier.

Headaches resulting from tension, particularly muscular tension in the neck, shoulders and upper back, may benefit from massage with the oils derived from neroli, rosemary, melissa, geranium (*Pelargonium*) and eucalyptus.

A swift emergency treatment when a headache threatens, as Virginia Clarkson of Streetly, West Midlands suggests, is to place two fingers from each hand on to the temples and press firmly.

See also Hangover (and related stomach upsets); Migraine.

Head lice and nits

Some reports estimate – but heaven knows who works out the figures – that three million Britons have head lice. Head lice are an unfussy lot and care not whether they live on adults' or children's hair. And they don't discriminate between clean and dirty hair – a simple shampoo will not shift them.

Nits are the tiny white shells from which baby lice have hatched. They stick to individual hairs and can be very difficult to remove, a fine-toothed comb being the preferred method.

In the past women waged war on head lice and nits with a variety of remedies, to cure them and then prevent their return. Dot Alsworth, now living in Oxfordshire, had her hair washed once a week, first with soap, then with vinegar, which was left on for several minutes, before rinsing it off, just in case she caught an infestation at school. Robert McElhinney from Horn Head in County Donegal remembers paraffin oil being put on to his hair.

Angela Moules, who is now ninety, was a nurse at Great Ormond Street Hospital for Sick Children in the 1930s and at the Postgraduate Medical School in Hammersmith during the Second World War. After the war she nursed in Germany with the charity Save the Children in a hospital near the Baltic. Angela's remedy for head lice was:

> *Oil of sassafras that was rubbed into the head, covered with lint and then dressed with a 'coppeline' bandage. The following day the head would be washed thoroughly.*

Angela says this remedy was wholly successful.

Carola Augustin suggests another remedy, and this one involves beer:

500 ml [17 fl oz] of milk
2 × 500 ml [17 fl oz] bottles of any kind of good beer
3 eggs
juice of 2 lemons
2 dessertspoons of vinegar

Mix all the ingredients together. Pour it over the head. Cover the hairline with cotton wool and carefully cover the hair with a plastic bag or cling film. Leave for at least half an hour. Then rinse the head well.

A herbal solution comes from Joannah Metcalfe's *Herbs and Aromatherapy* (1992):

20 drops geranium essence
40 drops bergamot essence
20 drops lavender essence
20 drops tea-tree oil
Add to 100 ml [3½ fl oz] of vegetable oil

Shake the blend before use. Massage blend thoroughly throughout the hair and scalp. Leave on for a minimum of one hour under cling film or a shower cap, or overnight if possible. Repeat the treatment four times over two days. Wash all bed linen, hats and cloths. The length of time the procedure is repeated is important. This helps ensure that the eggs as well as the insects are killed.

She also suggests that to wash the blend out of your hair, you should apply the shampoo first, before the water, otherwise the oil may prove stubborn.

Hiccups

There are some hilarious remedies for hiccups, which are actually spasmodic contractions of the diaphragm. Drinking from the other side of the glass sounds a little ridiculous, but some people insist it works. Another favourite remedy is to ask someone else to give the sufferer a fright. Provoking a sneeze with a feather or a pinch of snuff are other possible remedies, as is breathing in and out of a paper bag twenty times. An alternative is to hold your breath for a count of forty.

Most people ignore the problem because it usually resolves itself relatively quickly. If the hiccups become painful and continue over a long time a relaxant may be necessary, but this should be prescribed by a doctor. However, it might be worth trying this preparation suggested by Margaret Timms from Leamington Spa first:

> *Take 1 level teaspoon of sugar, drizzle vinegar on to the sugar until all the sugar is absorbed. Swallow quickly.*

Meanwhile, Virginia Clarkson from Streetly in the West Midlands recommends pinching your earlobes.

Immune system (boosting) ·

Some physicians will tell you that it is not possible to boost the immune system directly, but you can create the energy – with good diet and rest – that will enable the body to restore its own defence mechanisms. Our grandmothers seem to have recognised this by giving their families foods and remedies full of vitamins and minerals that were aimed at helping the body ward off infections.

One of the many tasks of national importance undertaken by members of the Women's Institute during the Second World War was to arrange the collection of rosehips. These were an excellent source of vitamin C for children living in the cities, since other fruits, such as lemons and oranges, were in short supply. (See pages 205-9 for more about the WI's extraordinary mission in collecting medicinal herbs.) Two teaspoons a day of rosehip syrup will help protect you against colds and flu, and here is an easy-to-make recipe adapted from Rachel Hunt's *The Wholefood Harvest Cookbook*:

2 lb [1 kg] ripe rosehips
4½ pints [2.6 litres] water
1 lb [500 g] demerara sugar

Wash and mince the rosehips. Bring the water to the boil in a large pan and add the rosehips. Bring back to the boil and simmer for 45 minutes. Allow to cool, then sieve through muslin or a jelly bag. Leave overnight to strain to make sure all the juice has run through. Return the juice to the pan and reduce the quantity by half by simmering. Add the sugar and simmer again until it has dissolved. Bring to the boil for a further five minutes. Pour into clean warm bottles.

*Cork or seal them tightly. The syrup will keep for only a few weeks
once opened, so it may be better to use small bottles.*

Linda Gray suggests a variation that doesn't use sugar and can be
drunk as a tea:

*Take one teaspoon of dried rosehips or one and a half teaspoons
of fresh, and mix with a pinch of ground cinnamon. Pour a cup
of freshly boiled water over the mixture and leave to stand for 10
minutes, then strain. Add a squeeze of lemon and, if needed, a little
honey to sweeten.*

Another famous remedy is malt extract with cod liver oil. This
comes again from the Women's Institute, appearing in its magazine
Home & Country, in February 1931.

*Malt extract with cod liver oil is one of the oldest and most
dependable remedies for deficiencies in diet and their attendant evils.
These are more in evidence at this time of year – in the change of
season – than at any other and they appear mostly as colds, coughs
and influenza.*

Cod liver oil has always been regarded as something of a cure-all in
itself. Originally it was taken in the fishing communities in Scotland
– and also in Norway and Iceland – to boost protection against
freezing weather. Gradually it became wider known for relieving
bone and joint complaints, and many children with rickets from
Victorian days onwards were duly given a daily dose. In more recent
times research has confirmed that cod liver oil and other oily fish are
rich in several essential fatty acids and are therefore beneficial, not

only for rheumatism and arthritis but also for the heart and circulatory systems.

Herbalist Anne McIntyre recommends a glycerite made with rosemary. Many glycerites do not use alcohol (see page 226), but this one does, and, Anne says, it makes a syrup with a kick and that the benefit comes from taking it every day.

Push as many sprigs of fresh rosemary as you can into a jar. Cover with 80 per cent glycerine and 20 per cent pure alcohol (brandy or vodka). Leave for two weeks, shaking the jar daily.

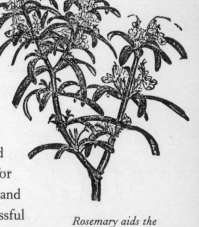

She adds: 'Rosemary is one of my favourite herbs. It represents eternal life. I use it a lot myself to help me be strong and to improve my memory. It also aids digestion and immunity, and helps the spirit and the mind. It can be used for headaches, migraine, to improve concentration and generally for depletion. Try and take a small glassful every day to get through the winter. It's very good for women on their own!'

Rosemary aids the immune system.

In central Europe beetroot has a reputation for aiding the immune system, and fresh, raw beetroot juice is given to convalescents. Like carrots, beetroot is also credited with having anti-cancer properties. Nutritionally, freshly boiled beetroot is better than the raw vegetable and is a good source of folate (folic acid), an essential nutrient for health.

In the Middles Ages the Welsh physicians from Myddfai took

prevention as seriously as cure. Here is their suggestion for 'taking care of yourself in seasons of changeable weather':

In this month [May] do not eat sheep's heads or trotters. Use warm drinks and take gentle emetics. Drink cold whey and the juice of fennel and wormwood.

Indigestion

If you're suffering from indigestion there's a great deal to be said for hot water, according to the traveller Annie Penfold (see page 209) and Ayurvedic practitioner Sebastian Pole. Sebastian points out that the digestive system is a little like a cooking pot. If you want to clean the pot, you do not use cold water that would solidify any grease, you would use warm water that melts the grease and washes it away. For this reason, drinking iced water is never advocated in Ayurvedic medicine.

The Egyptians, Greeks and Arab peoples all used rosemary to treat digestive problems and to aid what the French call *le transit intestinal*. Rosemary (*Rosmarinus*), with its antiseptic and tonifying properties, is still used in France to help reduce wind:

Take fresh sprigs of rosemary and make a tea or an infusion.

Tansy for gastric pain. The herb contains flavenoids, which help counteract intestinal spasms and so help flatulence. It is also renowned for helping to alleviate depression.

The physicians of Myddfai favoured tansy (*Tanacetum*), a flower that grew in most medieval gardens, and for gastric pain they suggested:

> Take a little tansy and reduce to a fine powder. Take with white wine and it will remove the pain.

Nicholas Culpepper, writing in 1653, concurs, stating:

> The decoction of the common tansy, or the juice drank in wine ... is also very profitable to dispel wind in the stomach, belly or bowels.

More recently Rachel Hunt, writing *The Wholefood Harvest Cookbook*, included one of her grandmother's recipes for ginger beer, which, she says, brings happy childhood memories. It is not only thirst-quenching but also, she adds, can help settle upset stomachs.

8 teaspoons sugar
¾ pint [450 ml] warm water
½ teaspoon fresh yeast
8 teaspoons ground ginger
12 oz [375 g] demerara sugar
1 pint [600 ml] boiling water
juice of 1 lemon
2½ pints [1.5 litres] cold water

> *Dissolve 1 teaspoon sugar in a little of the warm water. Stir in the yeast and leave to activate for 15 minutes. Add the rest of the water and 1 teaspoon ground ginger. Put into a large jar and*

cover with a piece of muslin. Then, every day for a week, add a tea-
spoon each of ginger and sugar. Dissolve the demerara sugar in the
boiling water. Add the lemon juice, cold water and the starter. Bottle
and cork – but not too tightly – and leave to ferment. Ginger beer can
be drunk after the third day.

A number of people have suggested taking a teaspoon of bicarbonate of soda in warm or hot water. An elderly friend of Jean Gardyne in Stroud finds this useful, while Cynthia Hawkins from nearby Cheltenham believes the same, saying: 'It's a bit kill or cure. If it is indigestion, it will cure it. If it really is nausea, then the drink will help you to be sick and subsequently feel better.'

Virginia Clarkson of Streetly in the West Midlands prefers to use:

one tablespoon of cider vinegar and one teaspoon of honey in a
glass or mug of hot water.

Other suggestions include taking milk. People with stomach ulcers are often advised to drink a glass of milk before a meal 'to line their stomach'. An alternative is to drink warm milk before bedtime to neutralise the acid.

In many parts of Europe it is possible to buy jars of raw potato juice, which is the traditional remedy for heartburn. The dosage is five to six dessertspoons of the juice before each meal to lessen reflux and burning. According to Linda Gray in her book *Traditional Remedies*, potato juice is a time-honoured way to relieve stomach cramps. This sounds as if it is more to do with the large intestine than the stomach. However, she points out that it is essential to avoid green potatoes, which are poisonous. Here is her recipe for making your own potato juice:

Peel and scrub half a pound [250 g] of potatoes and chop them into bite-sized pieces before putting them into a liquidiser or food processor. Add lemon juice to taste. Take two tablespoons before each meal but do not take for longer than 24 hours.

Dr Nick Read, medical adviser to the Gut Trust, suggests caution in using the lemon juice in this remedy. Although it might be fine in cases of stomach cramps, it could exacerbate heartburn.

Among the alternatives that Linda suggests are cabbage juice and the water in which new potatoes have been cooked.

Frances Wilkins from Habrough in northeast Lincolnshire remembers that her mother was a great believer in:

Sweet Nitre and Tincture of Rhubarb, which was mixed with hot water and a teaspoon of sugar.

She says it was a very reliable cure for stomach ache. 'It could be bought at the local chemist who sold everything and made up one's own recipe if wished.'

For a burning sensation that is likely to be reflux of stomach acids, a herbalist is likely to prescribe slippery elm (*Ulmus rubra*), which creates a slippery, soothing viscous coating on the inner digestive tract. The traditional way to take this is in a gruel:

one tablespoon of slippery elm powder mixed with hot water to make a paste. It can be flavoured with a little ginger, nutmeg or cinnamon.

Some herbalists will combine slippery elm with marshmallow. In her book *The Complete Floral Healer* Anne McIntyre states: 'Marshmallow is a wonderful remedy for any kind of irritation or inflammation inside or outside of the body, because of its great soothing and healing properties ... Marshmallow will help relieve heartburn and indigestion.'

Insect repellents

Several herbs are renowned as insect repellents, among them geranium (*Pelargonium*), lavender and mint. These would be hung in bunches or added to an oil, which would be drizzled on to pads or small cushions. Some herbs were dropped into water held in a small container over a candle, allowing the vapour to spread throughout the air.

Rue (*Ruta graveolens*), a strongly scented evergreen shrub, has many uses, ranging from relieving stomach cramps to inducing miscarriages. However, it is perhaps best known as an insect repellent and is especially effective against fleas. In the past it was customary for judges who were holding assize courts to have sprigs of rue on the bench to help combat the spread of pestilence and the possibility of gaol fever, which would be brought into the court by the prisoners from their terrible jails. Even now it is traditional in some courts for judges to be presented with posies of aromatic herbs. Another key herb in the judges' posies – and that of monarchs on Maundy Thursday, when they traditionally distribute alms to the poor – was thyme (*Thymus*), also renowned for its antiseptic properties.

The leaves and oil of rue are used in drinks, such as bitters, vermouth and grappa, but substances containing rue should never be applied directly to the skin because they can cause burning and blisters.

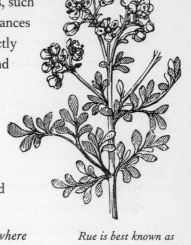

In the WI magazine *Home & Country* of October 1932, Mrs Smith reported that she had visited Sweden, and she had a suggestion that before travelling to any area where mosquitoes are present the traveller should prepare themselves:

> *Rub face, neck, wrists and ankles and anywhere else vulnerable with fifty:fifty salad oil and birch oil … It also smells nice and is very good for the skin.*

Rue is best known as an insect repellent.

Nowadays, herbalists are more likely to recommend oil of citronella. My mother, Joan Chappell, was a great believer in this substance and would duly anoint the entire family – including the dog – before any summer picnic or woodland walk. And I can confirm that none of us – not even the dog – suffered from any midge or horsefly bites during those outings.

Oil of citronella is an essential oil obtained from the leaves and stems of *Cymbopogon citratus* or, as it is more commonly known, lemon grass. It has strong anti-fungal properties as well as being used extensively as an insect repellent. In the United States it has been registered for this use since 1948.

For travellers to exotic, especially tropical, locations Kevin Allen, a dentist in Fulham, London, suggests that it is worth taking a good vitamin B supplement, containing both vitamins B6 and B12. Recent research shows that this will help stave off insect bites. He says: 'I've travelled widely in the developing world, and I believe it really helps. And even if it doesn't work for you insect-wise, this remedy won't do you any harm.'

Insomnia

Everyone has the odd night when it seems to be impossible to get to sleep. The mind is in overdrive or the body is restive. When sleep – or rather the lack of it – becomes a nightly battle, however, it becomes chronic insomnia. The number of people who experience insomnia at some point in their life is huge, and it affects all age groups.

The opium poppy (*Papaver somniferum*) was known from Neolithic times to have sleep-inducing properties, and in all the ancient civilisations it was used both to induce sleep and as an anaesthetic. It continued to be used for pain relief until the American Civil War (1861–5), after which morphine was more commonly used. In the eighteenth and nineteenth centuries opium – or its tincture, laudanum – became a recreational drug, but by then its highly addictive properties had been recognised.

As the Flopsy Bunnies found out in Beatrix Potter's tale, lettuce has a reputation for having a soporific effect. Both wild and cultivated lettuce contains a natural opiate called lectucarium, which has been referred to as having all the sedative effects of opium without the excitement. In the nineteenth century doctors and pharmacists would use lectucarium if opium was unavailable, the advantage being that lectucarium was not addictive. Lettuce is also a good source of vitamin C and contains hyoscyarnin, which is an anti-cramping agent.

Richard Clark-Monks of Chelsea, London, recommends lettuce sandwiches and a glass of hot milk or lettuce soup during the evening. The more traditional preparation is a decoction of lettuce seeds:

> *Boil half a litre [17 fl oz] of water. Add a tablespoon of lettuce seeds. Cover the saucepan or pot with a lid and simmer until the liquid is reduced to one-third.*

You can also make lettuce juice, adding a little lemon juice to give flavour.

Another ancient remedy is valerian (*Valeriana officinalis*), which has always been associated with restful sleep and relaxation. The name comes from the Latin *valere*, which means to be whole. Hippocrates is reputed to have used it in the fourth century BC, and it is also mentioned in Anglo-Saxon herbals. It was used to treat migraine, insomnia, hysteria and other nervous conditions, and it was in regular use as a sedative at the end of the First World War. It is in current use as a mild tranquilliser in Germany. Valerian root is available in the form of capsules and tinctures, but you can use the plant to make a tea. A Cornish friend suggests:

> *Just use half an ounce [15 g] of dried valerian root, add fresh mint leaves, and cover with boiling water. Leave to steep for at least one hour. Warm it again to drink.*

Valerian for insomnia.

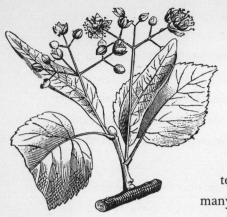

*Lime blossom
for insomnia.*

It is also interesting to note that valerian is the sovereign remedy for stage fright.

A number of other herbal teas have always been popular for treating insomnia, most particularly camomile and lime blossom. See page 223 for instructions on how to make herb teas and tisanes. Aniseed tea also has many supporters:

Boil 375 ml [13 fl oz] of water, add a teaspoon of aniseed, cover and simmer for 15 minutes. Strain before drinking it hot. You can add hot milk and also honey as a sweetener.

Hops (*Humulus*), a component of beer, have sedative properties too and a long history of use in cases of sleeplessness and restlessness, and some herbalists will combine hops with valerian. For mild cases of insomnia a hop pillow may be beneficial.

*Hops for mild
insomnia.*

Jellyfish stings

Jellyfish stings can be extremely painful, particularly if they are not treated quickly after the attack. With waters warming around the British coasts jellyfish are now increasingly regular visitors, including the Portuguese man-of-war. Kevin Allen, a much-travelled, London-based dentist, points out the value of vinegar for treating jellyfish stings:

> Pour vinegar on to a jellyfish sting. In Australia, where box jelly stings can be serious, if not fatal, vinegar is kept on all the beaches. But it works well for the UK variety too.

In coastal areas of the United States and South Africa a widespread folk remedy for jellyfish stings and insect bites is to apply meat tenderiser, an enzyme that helps break down the bonds between amino acids. For instant relief, though, many people recommend urine, dabbed on to the site of the sting.

Liver complaints

They say that the British are plagued by their bowels, while the French are preoccupied by their livers. The French have always sworn by good virgin olive oil, perhaps with a few drops of lemon juice, to stimulate a lazy liver, which is, of course, the body's detoxifying organ. This concoction should be taken daily and is thought to keep bad cholesterol at bay, too.

In France and throughout Mediterranean countries artichokes are also believed to balance the system. A French remedy suggests:

> *Do not throw away the water in which you have cooked artichokes but keep it to drink since it retains some of the beneficial qualities.*

Interestingly, the French and Swiss also recommend an infusion of artichokes for hepatitis, gout and rheumatism.

Dandelions (*Taraxacum officinale*) crop up in many different kinds of remedy. The traveller Annie Penfold (see page 209) recommends them for colds and coughs, and their diuretic and cleansing properties are advocated in the following remedy that occurs in both England and Wales:

> *Take four ounces [125 g] of fresh dandelion roots. Boil them in two pints [1.2 litres] of water until the liquid is reduced by half. Strain and drink a small glassful twice a day.*

The Oxford Book of Health Foods (2003) confirms that dandelion has been used in herbal medicine for many centuries, both in Europe and the East. One of the plant's common names is wet-the-bed (in French, *piss-en-lit*), and its root has been employed as a diuretic as well as a tonic, laxative and appetite stimulant. The root and leaves have been used to treat heartburn and flatulence, but its main usage has been in kidney and liver disorders.

In *A Modern Herbal* (1931) Mrs Grieve wrote: 'In hepatic complaints of persons long in warm climates, dandelion is said to afford very marked relief.' She recommended a broth made of sliced dandelion roots, stewed in boiling water with some sorrel leaves and an egg yolk. She suggests that this remedy should be taken daily for some months and adds that it 'has been known to cure seemingly intractable cases of chronic liver congestion'.

Mrs Grieve offers a further remedy using dandelion, which she calls a liver and kidney mixture:

> *Take one ounce [25 g] of broom tops, with half an ounce [15 g] of dandelion root boiled for 10 minutes in one and a half pints [900 ml] of water. The mixture is then strained and a small quantity of cayenne added. The dose should be one tablespoon, three times a day.*

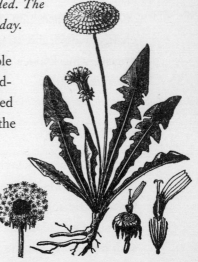

Dandelion acts as a diuretic.

Mrs Grieve also confirms that the humble apple helps the liver and counteracts the acidity of gout and indigestion. As we all learned as schoolchildren: 'An apple a day keeps the doctor away.' She points out that, through some innate instinct, we choose to eat an apple sauce with rich foods, such as pork and goose, and will often take a fresh apple with cheese.

Mastitis

Many women experience sore breasts just before their periods, and mastitis can also be due to an infection caused by bacteria entering the nipples, causing the breasts to become sore, swollen and even lumpy. Sometimes the lymph glands under the arms also swell.

Mrs Rotherham of south London recommends warm compresses:

> *Simply add a few drops of lavender, rose, geranium or camomile oil to warm water. Soak cloths and apply. This can be repeated up to four times a day.*

She adds that very gentle massage will stimulate lymph flow.

Another traditional solution is gentle massage using calendula cream, which is made from pot marigolds (*Calendula officinalis*). The tincture of marshmallow root (*Althaea officinalis*) added to a bath is also believed to relieve pain.

Another treatment, for which there seems no logic but that is clearly widely and strongly held, uses cabbage leaves to cover the breast. Anna Davies of south London is one of many women who subscribe to this.

Measles

May McElhinney, who is now in her seventies, was born and brought up in Carrickfinn, Kincasslagh in County Donegal, and she was given nettle soup after she developed measles when she was fifteen. The soup was reputed to bring out the rash, and May reports that her rash duly came out the following morning.

The Methodist John Wesley, in his book *Primitive Physick*, published in 1747, gives this advice for measles:

Immediately consult an honest Physician.

Drink only thin water-gruel, or milk and water, the more the better or toast and water.

If the cough be very troublesome, take frequently a spoonful of barley-water, sweetened with oil of sweet almonds newly drawn, mixed with syrup of maidenhair.

After the measles, take three or four purges, and for some weeks, take care of catching cold. Use light diet, and drink barley water instead of malt drink.

Barley water, made with pearl barley, has been used for centuries and was considered to be a nutritious baby food as well as useful for medicinal purposes. Possibly its benefit is that it is an easily absorbed source of carbohydrate, particularly for anyone unable to take solids. It is also soothing to both the digestive and urinary systems. Betty Browning from Coventry offers this recipe:

To make a simple barley water, simply wash one heaped tablespoon of barley, place in a pan with half a litre (or one pint) of water, bring to the boil, then simmer for half an hour. Strain and cool.

Barley water for many medicinal purposes.

Betty points out that often barley has been complemented by lemon. Here is her modern recipe for making lemon barley water:

Place 2 oz [50 g] of pearl barley into a sieve and pour over a kettleful of boiling water to clean it. Finely peel half a lemon,

removing only the outer waxy layer. Do not discard the lemon;
retain the juice for later use. Place the barley and lemon rind into a
saucepan and add 1 pint [600 ml] of water. Cover and simmer for
about 20 minutes. Strain. Add the lemon juice and one tablespoon
of sugar (to taste). Allow to cool before drinking.

Interestingly, lemon barley water is still the 'official' drink offered to tennis players at the Wimbledon Championships.

To make almond milk – which combines well with barley water – soak 2 oz (50 g) of whole almonds in warm water to help remove the skins. Pound them in a pestle and mortar or a modern food processor with 1½ pints (900 ml) of water. Make a paste, add up to a tablespoon of honey and strain through muslin.

Menopause

Menopause and menstruation (see page 116) are not, of course, illnesses or injuries, they are merely the normal functions of the female body. It is true that sometimes these functions are uncomfortable, if not downright painful or embarrassing – the hot flushes of menopause, for example – but they are entirely 'healthy'. Before over-the-counter solutions became available, our female forebears developed their own strategies.

In the Middle East and Indochina women were perhaps not quite so coy about menopause, seeing it as a rite of passage from child-bearing years to the time of wisdom and spirituality. The Chinese have herbal mixtures with delightful names, such as 'ease the journey'. In India the herb shatavari (*Asparagus racemosus*) is used for all phases of a woman's life, while a cup of pomegranate juice, with sugar to taste and a few drops of lime juice, is a sovereign remedy for hot flushes. Aloe vera is also prized as a remedy. In *Ayurvedic Medicine* Sebastian Pole states: 'It is a wonderful tonic for the female reproductive system. Its cooling and unctuous properties make it very effective for treating the hot and dry systems of menopause.'

In both the Far East and Middle East rosewater has always been rated highly to help with hot flushes, both when taken in a tea and as a delightful aromatic and cooling external spray.

In this country, along with lady's mantle (*Alchemilla xanthochlora*) – see more about this wonderful herb under Menstruation – sage (*Salvia*) is the standard remedy for night sweats and hot flushes, either as an extract or taken as an infusion. Modern trials have confirmed its value, and Maryon Stewart, author of *The Natural Menopause Kit*, recommends sage leaf. She also mentions two other traditional herbal remedies, St John's wort (*Hypericum perforatum*) as an anti-depressant and agnus castus (*Vitex agnus-castus*), which helps with mood swings. Marigold tea is also said to help hormonal imblances and hot flushes.

Sage for night sweats and hot flushes.

Red clover (*Trifolium pratense*) has been used traditionally as a herbal medicine for respiratory problems and chronic skin conditions, including eczema and psoriasis. It is also mentioned earlier as a blood cleanser. However, herbalists have always noted its affinity with women and have used it to treat conditions of the female reproductive system, both for heavy and painful periods and for the side effects of the menopause. Recently a research study has been launched into red clover as a natural alternative to allopathic (that is, pharmaceutical drug-based) hormone replacement therapy. In London Queen Charlotte's and Chelsea Hospital's menopause and PMS centre is carrying out a five-year study to see if red clover can reduce menopausal hot flushes.

In the West raspberry leaf also has a long pedigree of use both in pregnancy (see Morning sickness) and for menopausal problems if there is heavy bleeding, where its astringent properties may be valuable.

Menstruation

In Eastern medicine menstrual pain was combated by taking aloe vera gel three times a day for a week before a period was anticipated. The Indian name for aloe vera is *kumari*, meaning young maiden, which reveals its affinity for the female menstrual cycle.

For premenstrual bloating lovage (*Levisticum officinale*) – a form of wild celery originally from mountainous areas of the Mediterranean – makes a useful tea that helps reduce water retention:

> *Place a heaped teaspoon of fresh chopped lovage leaves and roots in a cup and cover with boiling water. Allow to steep for five to ten minutes and strain. Add honey to taste.*

From medieval times onwards in Europe, the herb lady's mantle (*Alchemilla xanthochlora*) was considered 'a woman's best friend', and some modern herbalists still promote it and its close relative

A. alpina. It is reputed to be of use to women with heavy periods and period pain by helping to stimulate menstrual flow. It can be used as a tonic after childbirth or miscarriage and for any gynaecological infection.

Lady's mantle can also be made into a wash to help 'feminine itching'. Here's a lotion recipe from Linda Gray's *Traditional Remedies*:

> *Soak a handful of lady's mantle in 1 cup of rosewater overnight. Strain through coffee filter paper and bathe the skin gently, twice a day.*

Pamela Jackson from Basingstoke remembers that her great-aunt told her that if her 'private parts' were sore or irritated she should take a leaf of houseleek (*Sempervivum*), break it in half and gently rub the infected area with it. It's indeed possible that this would have worked. Culpeper rated houseleek for 'hot inflammations', claiming that it 'cools and tempers the blood and spirits'. Dr Henry Oakeley, a Fellow of the Royal College of Physicians, confirms that houseleek is refrigerant, astringent and diuretic, and he points out that the bruised leaves of the fresh plant, or its juice, are often applied as a poultice to burns, scalds, contusions, scrofulous ulcers and in inflammatory conditions of the skin, when it generally gives immediate relief.

The medieval physicians of Myddfai wrote in praise of leeks:

> *The juice is good against the vomiting of blood. It is good for women who desire children to eat leeks.*

They added:

> *Take leeks and wine to cure the bite of adders and venomous beasts.*

Migraine

The causes of migraine are unclear, although many people, through trial and error, find their personal trigger and therefore a way to manage their attacks. Some migraines seem to be related to diet, but stress also, clearly, plays a part.

Margaret Paxton, who now lives in Knaresborough, Yorkshire, spent her childhood in Cumbria, and she remembers how her grandmother suffered from migraines and how her son would cycle over to give her something that would take away the pain. He would toast bread over the fire until he had crumbs, then he would add water, salt and pepper and his mother would sip the mixture from a spoon. It's hard to know how this preparation helped, although possibly it settled her stomach. It's interesting that some people swear by carbon from burned toast as a remedy for hangovers. The theory – not borne out scientifically – is that the carbon acts as a kind of filter.

Less surprising is the use of ginger to offset the nausea associated with migraine. Migraine Action, the charity that offers help to people afflicted with migraines, states of ginger that 'there is evidence of efficacy in preventing attacks'. It also recommends four to six fresh leaves of feverfew (*Tanacetum parthenium*) or 50 mg of the dried leaves daily. *See also* Headaches.

Ginger to offset nausea.

Morning sickness

There are surprisingly few remedies for this most common of conditions in pregnancy. Ginger tea and ginger cordial have been suggested, and these remedies are likely to have some validity because ginger has been used for centuries for calming motion and travel sickness. It is warming and pungent and therefore settles the stomach, soothes indigestion and dispels flatulence. Here is a traditional remedy for making ginger cordial:

1 oz [25 g] ginger root, bruised
8 oz [250 g] granulated sugar
1 teaspoon tartaric acid
½ lemon, sliced

Place all the above ingredients into a bowl and cover with 4 pints [2.5 litres] of boiling water. Stir until the sugar has dissolved, then cover and allow to stand for three to four days. Strain the liquid through muslin, pour into bottles and seal tightly. Leave for several days before drinking the cordial.

The excessive use of this remedy should be avoided.

Raspberry leaves are recalled by some older women, and the Rev. Canon Celia Thomson at Gloucester Cathedral offers this recipe for raspberry leaf tea:

In the early days of pregnancy, take dried raspberry leaves and make a tea, tisane or infusion.

Raspberry leaves for morning sickness.

It's not just the leaves of raspberries that were thought to be beneficial, and Cynthia Swift, who now lives in La Curano, Spain, remembers how, half a century ago, she was given wild raspberries to help 'ease' childbirth.

Mosquito and midge bites

If the insect repellents (on page 104) have failed and you've been bitten, there is the old country remedy of rubbing the site with dock (*Rumex*) leaves, also used, of course, if you have been stung with nettles. Dabbing the bite with witch hazel, which is astringent and has some anti-inflammatory properties, is an old-fashioned solution, as is using essence of lavender in the same way. Some people recommend rubbing the bite with a spring onion.

Adele Murray from Dumfries and Galloway suggests using an aspirin:

> *Take an aspirin tablet and add a little water, so it becomes a paste. Apply the paste directly on to the mosquito bite. It works for midges too. We have lots of both in Scotland! I have a friend who swears by this.*

Possibly this second remedy, from an unidentified source, has its roots in Scotland too:

> *Apply whisky to the bites to reduce swelling.*

A more cosmetic solution comes from an issue of the Women's Institute magazine *Home & Country* from September 1932:

> *To stop the itching overnight, cover the spot with a thick layer of*

cold cream; powder it with talc till it looks quite dry, cover with fine linen.

A lotion made with camomile may also be soothing. The above remedies are only applicable to the British types of mosquito or midge. Travellers to areas where mosquitoes and other insects may carry serious diseases, such as malaria and yellow fever, have obviously required other solutions and nowadays are usually immunised in advance of their trip.

A few years ago I became badly bitten on a trip to Australia, where the very many insects clearly enjoyed a drop of British blood. My friend, Kae Chapman-Turner, treated me with a solution of cloudy ammonia, dabbed on to all the bite sites. This rather fierce substance, which is normally used for cleaning everything from your jewellery to the inside of the freezer, made sure that any eggs laid by an insect under the skin would be sterilised and not hatch out. It seemed a very reasonable course of action at the time.

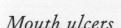

Camomile for mosquito and midge bites.

Mouth ulcers

Mouth ulcers can be very painful, and most of the remedies that have been remembered aimed at soothing the problem. Chewing a stick of liquorice root can help, and it will freshen your mouth at the same time. If you're not a fan of liquorice, you could try making a herbal gargle. As for sore throats, rosemary tea has always been a favourite remedy, but thyme, lemon balm, nettle or camomile can also be used.

Other traditional remedies include using a mouthwash made with tincture of myrrh, which has antiseptic properties. Here is a variation given by an aromatherapist:

> *Add two drops of myrrh, two of tea-tree oil, and a teaspoon of sea salt in a glass of water. Stir to dissolve the salt. Swill the mouthwash around thoroughly. This combination will both soothe and speed up healing.*

Myrrh is a resin derived from the sap of the tree *Commiphora myrrha*, which is native to eastern and western Africa, the Middle East, South America and the West Indies. In the story of the Nativity myrrh, alongside gold and frankincense, was one of the gifts the Magi, or three wise men, offered to the infant Jesus. At that time myrrh was more rare and precious than frankincense. The ancient Egyptians used it in the process of embalming, and it was a constituent of the Jews' holy oil. In ancient Rome – where it was five times the cost of frankincense – it was burned at funerals to mask the smell of burning corpses.

Myrrh has long been sought after for use in the making of perfumes and cosmetics, but it also has a reputation for making an effective mouthwash to treat soft gums and ulcerating throats. It is still used today in mouthwashes, toothpowders and also, since it is anti-fungal, to treat athlete's foot. In the Ayurvedic tradition it is used for a wide variety of treatments, including congestive heart disorders and 'scraping' cholesterol out of the system; painful periods in women; externally to repair broken bones and bruising; and, as in the West, as the first line in the treatment of mouth ulcers and cold sores, and in fungal conditions.

Nappy rash

Jeanette Watson moved from her native Scotland to New Zealand in the 1960s. Since then she has passed on to numerous young mothers in New Zealand a remedy for nappy rash that was given to her by her midwife in Paisley more than forty years ago.

After washing and drying the baby's bottom, apply the white of a raw egg to the area of the rash. Ensure your hand is clean. Let the baby have a few minutes kicking free, this to allow the egg white to dry, and then put on his clean nappy. Repeat this each time you change the nappy.

See also Bedsores.

Night sight and sight deficiencies

Many British children have been encouraged to eat carrots so they could 'see in the dark'. In fact, this is not an old wives' tale but has a basis in sound scientific fact. Carrots are rich in beta-carotene, which the body converts into vitamin A. It is a deficiency in this vitamin that causes poor night vision and also sore eyes.

Until Tudor times, and probably beyond, vitamin A deficiency was prevalent in a large proportion of the population, which perhaps goes some way to explain the common idea that certain wells and springs – whose water supply may have been rich in minerals that would counteract this deficiency – would offer relief for blindness and other eye conditions. Throughout the world there are springs and wells that are meant to bring health benefits – if not miraculous cures – and so have developed an aura of mystery and holiness. Sometimes a water source's reputation was purely local, in other instances centres of healing grew up around the well or spring, along with myriad myths, superstitions and sacred ceremonies.

Some of these are thought to date back to the Celts of pre-Roman times, who would throw votive offerings of ceremonial swords, small statues and precious jewellery into rivers and lakes. Pre-Christian holy wells, which offered both physical and spiritual healing, often had Celtic legends attached to them and with attendant 'guardians'. Believers would tie offerings – known as clooties – to nearby trees or shrubs, and sometimes wooden carvings of a damaged limb or organ would be tossed into the well.

In *A Celtic Book of Days* Sarah Costley and Charles Knightly suggest that Beltane, the first day or the first Sunday in May, is the best time to visit holy wells: 'Before using the water, be sure to throw in a silver coin, pin or other suitable offering; insulting the well by leaving rubbish may cause it to dry up or move away. After drinking, tie a rag torn from your clothing to a nearby bush; anyone who dares to remove such offerings will take your troubles or sickness with them.'

The early Christian Church, which understood that people would not readily set aside their faith in cures from sacred wells, promptly 'Christened' them, usually with the names of women saints. The sites were used mainly by local people, and the usage continued until surprisingly recently. For example, water from Eye-well in Market Lavington, Wiltshire, was being collected as late as the 1940s to treat an old woman suffering from cataracts.

See also Eyes (tired and sore).

Nosebleeds

There is an old wives' tale about slipping a key or keys down the back of the neck to help cure a nosebleed. This may cause the patient to shiver and so contract blood vessels – possibly those that were causing the bleeding – but it sounds rather a long shot.

There are other traditional remedies that would seem to be more effective. My mother would recommend pinching the nose tightly with the thumb and index finger, just as if you were about to go underwater. This pressure had to be maintained for five or more minutes, and it was followed by a cold compress on the forehead and nose.

A childhood friend's mother, Nora Smith, would tell us to sniff cold water, then very gently blow the nose so that any remaining blood clot could be expelled.

Frequent or long-lasting nosebleeds should be reported to a doctor, because in some instances high blood pressure or other underlying conditions may be the cause.

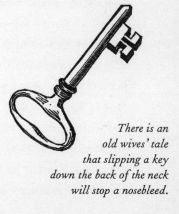

There is an old wives' tale that slipping a key down the back of the neck will stop a nosebleed.

Osteoarthritis

O It would be cruel to suggest that there is any kind of cure for arthritis, but people have come up with remedies that may help to alleviate some of the symptoms and relieve some of the pain.

One of the quainter – and perhaps slightly worrying – remedies that has been suggested is the use of a patent lubricant called WD-40. Eileen Blenkinsop from Doncaster frequently has crippling pain from arthritis. One day, in sheer desperation, she rubbed some WD-40 into her shoulder. To her amazement, she experienced almost instant relief and so promptly tried it on her fingers with the same happy result. She wondered if she was unique in this experience, but when she wrote to the company that makes the product she learned that every week they receive a number of letters from other arthritis sufferers claiming relief. The company is rightly extremely cautious about these claims and points out that, while the lubricant has a huge number of uses, it was not designed for use on the human body and has not been medically tested.

Jo Cumming, who heads the helpline at Arthritis Care, the national charity for people with arthritis, would certainly not recommend this remedy. However, she does suggest one treatment that may offer comfort and benefit in some forms of arthritis, particularly osteoarthritis – wheatbags. These are available in various shapes and sizes, and are not always filled with wheat. Simply pop a wheatbag in the microwave for between 20 and 30 seconds – or a conventional oven for much longer – and then place it against the affected area. Jo has an excellent household tip to add to this remedy: wheatbags can smell a bit mouldy after a while, but a few drops of essential oil, especially lavender, will overcome the problem.

Jo also discovered a continental alternative to the wheatbag. During a recent trip to Belgium she found that cherry stones were widely used in bags. The stones, usually a by-product of commercial or home jam-making, are cleaned and dried and put into little fabric bags. They can then be microwaved or wrapped in foil or put in a pot with a lid and heated in the oven.

Another home remedy that uses heat to soothe arthritic joints has been suggested by Jean Rogerson, who used to be a nurse at the former Bolton District General Hospital:

> *We would make wax baths, just with melted wax, for people with arthritis in their hands and feet. The patients would dip their hands and feet into the wax a couple of times, and the wax would set on to them, holding in the heat. Then when the wax had cooled, we would simply peel it off.*

As well as external treatments, some remedies to be taken internally have been recommended. One is to drink a glass of cider vinegar every morning, although there is no clinical evidence to indicate that this is valuable. Another, which has been a tradition for many years, suggests that people with arthritis should drink cabbage water. Here is a verse, 'The Pudding Lady', which is 'an extract from lines by a member of Whittinton Women's Institute after a talk by Miss Petty, May 1931'.

> *For all the ills that flesh is heir to,*
> *Be they great or be they small,*

There's a cure if but you care to
Cook your vegetables all,
As the 'Pudding Lady' tells you,
When she lectures in your hall.

Are you old or are you ailing?
Do your joints rheumatic creak?
There's a remedy unfailing
And it is not far to seek:
You need only quaff the water
From your cabbage week by week.

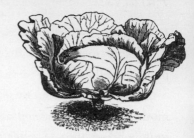

Cabbage water for
osteoarthritis.

Interestingly, poultices made from cabbage leaves have also been suggested to give relief to rheumatic joints.

A practical suggestion from Althea Wilson in Chelsea is that the best thing one can do for stiff and painful joints is to keep moving and find a suitable form of exercise. She has a childhood memory of an old lady who loved gardening but had arthritic knees, and she used to kneel down carefully on a hot water bottle to do those low-level garden chores. She also recalls hearing how people were advised to take up knitting for at least ten minutes a day if they had arthritis in their hands and fingers. In severe cases, people would use very large, wooden needles.

There has been a custom of people with arthritis wearing copper or 'magnetic' bracelets. There is no scientific explanation for this, and claims that the magnets work on the traces of iron in the blood are completely unfounded. There is the possibility that some minute trace elements of copper may be absorbed through the skin, but there's not much evidence that these are of benefit.

Paralysis

It was only in the 1950s that a vaccine against poliomyelitis was found and made generally available. Before that, paralysis from polio and other diseases was not uncommon.

Janet Stubbins from Wookey Hole, Somerset, recounts how her mother became paralysed after a bad fever at the age of five. Her grandmother, Julia Hatcher, was advised by a passing gypsy to treat the little girl with massage using an oil made from snails. As Janet points out, around Wells and in the Mendip Hills snails live abundantly in the drystone walls. She adds: 'They are still collected even now and eaten by a lot of country folk. You put them in salt water to kill them, clean them (twice) and boil them, removing the shells with a pin.'

The gypsy's snail massage oil remedy was to place snails in a sealed jar and bury it in the garden for a few months. The snails died and eventually became an oil that was poured out of the jar, leaving the snail shells behind. After three or four months of massage, Janet's mother started to walk again and returned to school. And she lived to be ninety-three.

Patient care

Like many women over the centuries, Betty Smith's grandmother, Lily Elliott (Pownall by a later marriage), kept a little notebook of her favourite remedies and recipes. Many of these books and notes have been lost, but fortunately Betty, who is in her mid-eighties and lives in Devon, has carefully preserved this notebook. It probably dates from 1870–80 and contains recipes for everything from lemon tart to cough mixture. One remedy is called 'An aromatic vinegar cooling lotion for the sick room'. Betty believes her grandmother would have used this to clean and refresh both the patient and the room itself. The recipe is:

Handful of rosemary
Handful of wormwood
Handful of lavender
Handful of mint

Put the herbs into a large stone jar. Add one gallon [4.5 litres] of strong vinegar. Cover the jar closely and leave by the fire for four days. Strain and add one ounce [25g] of camphor powder. Bottle and seal it.

Marjorie Melville, who was in service in Scotland in the nineteenth century, also kept a collection of remedies that have been passed down to her granddaughter, Anne Bisset. Marjorie's remedy for a simple disinfectant was:

Cut 2 or 3 good-sized onions in halves and place them on a plate on the floor. They absorb noxious effluae in the sick room in an incredibly short time and are greatly to be preferred to perfumery for the same purpose. They should be changed every six hours.

In order to prevent infection from spreading, she recommended:

Burn a piece of saltpetre the size of a walnut in every room wherein there is an infectious disease, also drink water in which a small piece of saltpetre has been dissolved.

Hyssop (*Hyssopus*) has been used since early times to cleanse the air and, as a medicinal remedy, to treat chest problems such as catarrh and bronchitis. It is mentioned a number of times in the Bible, probably because it was considered a holy herb, used to cleanse sacred places, and was also believed to help lepers. David refers to it in Psalm 51:7: 'Purge me with hyssop, and I shall be clean; wash me and I shall be whiter than snow.' In the seventeenth century,

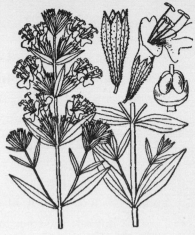

Hyssop to cleanse the air and treat chest problems.

and possibly before, it was used with a mixture of either honey or figs to kill worms and act as a laxative. It is the source of the essential oil camphor.

Rheumatism (rheumatoid arthritis)

r As with osteoarthritis, most remedies are able only to alleviate briefly the all too painful symptoms of this condition, they are unlikely to effect any kind of cure. Both forms of arthritis are degenerative conditions, gradually eroding the joints. In a small percentage of cases, the disease can be 'switched off' by adaptations to the diet, but as consultant physician Dr Gail Darlington, who has done a lot of research in this area, points out, dietary changes make little difference in about 60 per cent of cases.

Many unlikely remedies turn out – with considerations and sometimes appropriate warnings as well – to have positive benefits for some patients. Marie Thomson tells the following tale: 'In the 1960s, when my husband was posted abroad, we let our house to an Austrian lady called Mrs Ayres (as far as I can remember). She came to see us and asked if she could bring her beehives with her. We agreed. We only found out later, knowing nothing about bees, that this was a big mistake. We fell out with all the neighbours, the grass-cutting people refused to come, and it cost us to have the swarms re-housed when the bees refused to leave when we returned.

'To cut a long story short, I asked

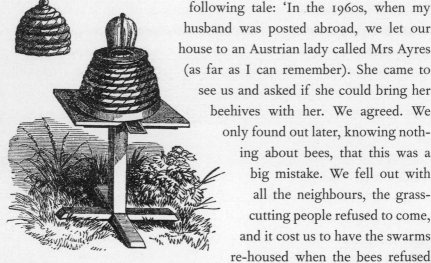

Bee stings for rheumatism.

Mrs Ayres what she did with the honey, but she told me she wasn't interested in the honey, only the bees. I thought she must be a doctor because she kept referring to her patients, but she told me she treated people for arthritis with bee stings to the back. She had some famous clients, including Robert Helpmann, the ballet dancer, and Jack Warner, the actor of *Blue Lamp* fame. She seemed quite genuine, because some years later I heard Jack Warner speak on the radio about her, saying how she had completely changed his life. He could hardly get out of the chair before she treated him (in our house I might add). He said it hurt at the time but it was worth it.

'I mentioned this remedy to my mother who was in her seventies at the time, but she had never heard of it, but my grandmother who was in her nineties told me it was a well-known fact in her youth that bee stings cured arthritis.'

The bee stings would not effect a cure but, because the substance in the sting is believed to contain anti-inflammatory agents, it may relieve the pain, stiffness and swelling of arthritis. There has been – and there continues to be – some research conducted in various parts of the world into the effectiveness of honey bee venom, also known as apitherapy. Obviously any patient contemplating this route must be cautioned that there are people in whom a bee sting causes a severe allergic reaction, which could even be fatal.

However, the benefit seems to have been documented in some patients, although bee stings are neither pleasant nor easy to administer. Apitherapy is also being tested for its value in treating multiple sclerosis.

Mary Wilson from Melrose in Roxburghshire has a remedy that

sounds equally painful. Now in her eighties, Mary learned from her mother to:

Nettles for rheumatism.

> *Gather a small bunch of stinging nettles, before the flowering season, and to use them to beat the area of rheumatism, be it an arm or leg.*

She says that the area may then itch for a day or two but the pain will have gone. 'The stinging sensation is not nearly so bad as the rheumatic pain,' she insists. Dr Darlington points out that nettles may contain some quantity of histamine, which explains this phenomenon, and according to Peter Cooper, who wrote nature notes for parish magazines in Cornwall, ointments were often made from the leaves of nettles to relieve rheumatism.

Another Scottish remedy comes from Colin McLeod of Dundee. He found this when he was clearing the effects of his aunt's house but believes it dates back to his grandparents' times, probably sometime in the nineteenth century.

> *½ pint [300 ml] white wine vinegar*
> *½ pint [300 ml] turpentine*
> *¼ pint [150 ml] methylated spirits*
> *½ oz [15 g] Opodeldre*
> *2 drachms camphor*
> *2 yolks of fresh eggs (not the white)*

> *Dissolve the Camphor in the Methylated Spirits. Beat up the Yolks and mix with the Vinegar and turpentine, then shake well up*

together and then add all the other parts.
POISON: *For external use only. Rub the affected parts.*

Peter Homan of the Royal Pharmaceutical Society of Great Britain suggests that the 'Opodeldre' mentioned here is probably opodeldoc, a liniment made with soft soap, camphor, rosemary oil, water and alcohol. It was used to rub on rheumatism, sore muscles and sprains.

A similar remedy appears on the website www.a-day-in-the-life.powys.org.uk, which contrasts the lifestyles of 1891 and of the present day in Powys, Wales. A handwritten embrocation for rheumatism, sprains and bruises calls for equal parts of opodeldoc, camphorated oil, camphorated spirits (of) wine, rectified spirits (of) turpentine and spirits (of) hartshorn. It suggested the addition of 'laudanum enough to tinge the above with a yellowish hue' and again it was clearly marked 'Poison'.

Jenny Kelly from Cornwall recommends the following linctus:

Marinade four large heads of garlic in four-fifths of a pint [480 ml] of brandy for 10 days. Take half a teaspoon in half a glass of water first thing in the morning.

While for relief, she suggests:

Mix together 2 oz [50 ml] of olive oil and 2 oz [50 ml] of surgical spirit and massage into the affected joints for 15 minutes night and morning.

Dr Vivien Martin from Worthing also suggests a rub:

Grate fresh ginger into sesame oil and rub it into the skin.

Skin diseases

The skin is the body's largest organ, and the Chinese in particular have always taken skin diseases very seriously. In their traditional herbal medicine there are very particular herbs that aid psoriasis and eczema, but the precise combination of ingredients differs to suit the constitution of the sufferer.

In Britain the walnut tree (*Juglans regia*) has provided both an infusion and a lotion to benefit scrofulous diseases, herpes and eczema. Mrs Grieve in *A Modern Herbal* (1931) suggests taking one ounce (25 g) of dried bark or leaves (but slightly more if using fresh leaves) to one pint (600 ml) of standing water. This must be allowed to stand for six hours before straining the liquid off. It should then be taken in wineglassful doses, three times a day. Mrs Grieve adds that the same infusion can also be employed at the same time for outward application. She advises that you should gather the leaves only in fine weather, in the morning, after the dew has been dried by the sun. 'The prevalence of an east wind is favourable, as dry air facilitates the process of drying. Reject all stained leaves.'

Hildegard of Bingen, the medieval mystic and healer (see pages 182–6) suggested another tree-based remedy for skin disorders:

Crush cherry seeds and mix with bear fat to make a paste and apply externally.

In medieval Wales the physicians of Myddfai offered a remedy specifically for 'dry scurvy disease of the eyelids':

Take strawberry juice, hen's fat and May butter, pound them well together and keep in a horn box. Anoint thine eyelids well before going to bed.

Finding a reliable source of bear fat and May butter may prove a challenge nowadays. Easier to find are stinging nettles (*Urtica dioica*) which, when made into a soup or a tea, have long been reputed to help eczema. A lotion can also be made with nettles for eczema and also to help dandruff. It is recommended that you should wear gloves when you are picking and preparing them. Rinse first, then discard any tough stalks before steaming or boiling the leaves and soft stems.

The herbalist Anne McIntyre believes in fresh coriander (*Coriandrum sativum*). 'I was staying in the mountains of Columbia for a time, and every day we had breakfast of potato soup served with fresh coriander. It was the first time I had tasted it. It is amazing for the digestion, and it helps you stay level-headed. I recommend it for allergies, hot flushes and skin conditions where there is heat. In Ayurveda it is used for eczema and urticaria. I use the seeds a lot too.'

Coriander for eczema and urticaria.

Camomile (*Chamaemelum*) has been used medicinally since ancient times and has been prescribed by physicians from all the great civilisations. It has been – and continues to be – used for skin inflammations because of its anti-inflammatory and antiseptic properties. It has been used for ointments, creams and lotions to treat everything from nappy rash to sore gums. A number of studies have confirmed its efficacy for skins conditions, used both externally and internally.

Here is an infusion from Janet Mead in Coventry that combines camomile with mallow (*Malva*) and lemon verbena (*Aloysia triphylla*), also known for their skin calming qualities.

1 teaspoon dried camomile
1 teaspoon dried lemon verbena
1 teaspoon mallow petals
sugar or honey to taste

Rinse out a teapot in hot water, and put in the dried herbs. Add 3 cups of boiling water, cover and steep for five minutes. Strain into cups and serve immediately, with a little sugar or honey to taste.

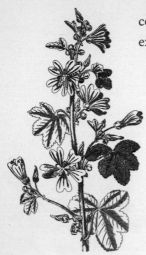

Mallow combined with other ingredients can help calm the skin.

For external use, cucumber, grated until it is semi-liquid, can be gently massaged into an inflamed area. It is said to be cooling.

Splinters

An extraordinary number of people have suggested that a mixture of soap and sugar is an old-fashioned but effective treatment for splinters and infected fingers. According to Pam Davison, who comes from Darlington, County Durham, a mixture of ordinary soap and sugar mixed together and piled on to a small pad would 'draw out' anything lodged in the skin. A remedy from her childhood, she used this for her own children, who are now in their forties. She has also used this remedy for boils and abscesses. Sheena McClay, who now lives in New Jersey in the USA, recalls the same remedy from when she was growing up on the Isle of Bute.

If we had a splinter, Mum would cut a small piece of soap and add some sugar, blend it together and apply it to the splinter (or skelf as we called it in Scotland), and within hours the skin would soften up so much that the skelf would come out easily.'

Gwladys Townesend from southeast London also kept a personal book of household hints and remedies, which her granddaughter, Hazel Townesend, believes may date from just after the First World War. Gwladys wrote:

When a splinter has been driven into the hand it can be extracted without pain with steam. Nearly fill a wide-mouthed bottle with hot water and place the hand over the mouth of the bottle, and press lightly. The suction will draw the flesh down and in a minute or two the steam will extricate the splinter and also the inflammation.

Here is a preparation from the 1920s or 1930s that uses flour and castor oil. It was recorded by Mrs Shapland from Chulmleigh in north Devon.

Make a paste of flour and castor oil. Put the paste around the affected finger or hand and leave for 12 hours, then the splinter will come out easily.

The Ayurvedic practitioner Sebastian Pole says that 'castor oil has renowned drawing properties'.

Sprains

In *A Modern Herbal* (1931) Mrs Grieve recommended leaves from the elder tree (*Sambucus*) as an ointment for sprains, bruises and chilblains. She gives a remedy that consists of taking three parts of fresh elder leaves to four parts of lard and two of prepared suet. The elder leaves must be heated with the melted lard and suet until the colour is extracted, then strained through a linen cloth under pressure and allowed to cool. She adds that the same mixture, with the addition of a little linseed, can be applied to haemorrhoids (piles).

Many parts of the elder are used in herbal medicine, including the bark, leaves, buds, flowers and berries. The bark has been used as a strong purgative since the days of Hippocrates; the leaves are used to make an ointment for sprains and bruises; and the flowers and berries are made into teas, lotions and wines. Elder has even been described as 'the medicine chest of country people'.

Mrs H. from Bakewell in Derbyshire, who is now in her mid-nineties, reports that the most used herb in her childhood home was comfrey (*Symphytum officinale*). She recommends it for sore feet and also for sprains.

> *For sprains of the wrists, and ankles, the broad comfrey leaves were soaked in hot water and laid on a hot towel or flannel and used as a compress.*

She says she grows comfrey in her garden even now and still uses it.

Taki Jaffer from Portsmouth suggests that an egg-white paste is hugely effective. He says: 'I sprained my wrist playing squash not long ago and this worked for me.'

Make a paste of egg whites, turmeric and salt. The paste sticks
like glue to the sprained joint, holding the muscles and ligaments in
place. After several days, there will be a real improvement.

Turmeric and salt are also used in this traditional Indian remedy, which has been recommended by Naina Ardeshani from Coventry. She mixes three parts of turmeric to one part salt to make a paste for sprains, omitting the egg whites mentioned above and using a binding or bandage instead. She applies the paste as hot as the skin can take it and adds a hot water bottle to help retain the heat as the paste starts to cool. She warns that turmeric is a dye that will mark both skin and, even more permanently, any clothing that it touches.

Here's a liniment for strained muscles and sprains that uses oils. The provenance is unknown, but it possibly originated in North America:

½ oz [15 g] lobelia oil
½ oz [15 g] St John's Wort oil
½ oz [15 g] wormwood oil
1 tablespoon ginger oil
1 tablespoon cayenne oil

Mix all the ingredients and massage three times daily.

In her *Tried Favourites Cookery Book* Mrs Kirk suggests a mustard lotion:

Mix 2 oz [50 g] mustard with ½ pint [300 ml] spirits of wine and
2 drachms of camphor; let it stand 3 days in a bottle carefully corked,
then strain it off, and keep closely bottled for use.

Stiff necks and swollen glands

When she was a child Elma Roberts from Pentre in Mid-Glamorgan always seemed to have swollen glands. Even now she occasionally has a 'lump' behind her ear. Her grandfather had his own method of treatment for many ailments, and Elma says that a doctor was never called in or consulted. The treatment for the swollen glands was a salt bag, which was warmed in the oven before she held it against her neck. Elma used the same treatment on her daughters if they had minor neck problems and even now she keeps a salt bag for her own use. She says: 'I don't know if it is the right thing to do but it is comforting and seems to reduce the swelling and discomfort.'

A variation of this comes from Joan Griffiths of Huntington, Cheshire, who recounts how her grandmother in Liverpool would take a large potato, boil it until it was soft and then place it in a long woollen sock. It was then mashed until it became a poultice for the patient's or – as Joan put it – victim's neck.

See also Throats (sore).

Stress

Our grandmothers' generation was largely unfamiliar with the term 'stress', certainly as it is commonly used today, with its connotations of personal anxiety, work-linked pressures, emotional turmoil and physical exhaustion. For writers and musicians, the word was used to imply emphasis – stressing a word, a phrase or a note. An architect or orthopaedic surgeon might use the term in reference to structural stress – of a building or a bone fracture.

It was only in the early part of the twentieth century that Sigmund Freud and his followers 'discovered' the subconscious mind and its impact on human behaviour and wellbeing, and it was really in the dreadful aftermath of the First World War, when there were thousands of shell-shocked and traumatised young men returning home, that doctors were alerted to the realities of genuine stress and its impact on long-term health.

Nowadays, some young people seem to assume that you cannot be working hard enough if you are not completely 'stressed out'. It has almost become a fashion item and is regarded as the source of many of our ills. Sadly, due in a large part to the speed with which we now live our lives and our high expectation of material comfort, it is, indeed, endemic.

This is not to say that there were not day-to-day stress factors (as we now call them) in our grandmothers' lives. After all, they also endured bereavement, family and financial crises, long working hours and few holidays, as well as wars, terrorism and financial recessions. They might have suggested that someone was suffering 'from their nerves', even to the point of nervous exhaustion. Extreme cases might have been referred to as 'hysteria'. But it wasn't seen as a specific condition to which most people were subject, by way of coping with their everyday existence.

As a result, there are not many old remedies that are purely for engendering calmness and relaxation. One infusion, suggested by Judy Townsend of Stratford-upon-Avon, uses lovely, calming lavender:

> *Take a sprig of lavender about three or four inches long. Place it into a mug or cup and add very hot water – just off the boil. Allow*

it to steep for five minutes with a saucer balanced on the top of the cup. Leave the lavender sprig in place as you sip it. It really does make you relax.

Cherries to help combat mental fatigue.

Lavender was also used in the bedroom, again for its relaxing qualities, with a few drops of essential oil on a pillow to aid sleep. It is also one of the few essential oils that can safely be applied directly on to the skin.

Other herbs recommended for helping anxiety and depression include borage (*Borago officinalis*), vervain (*Verbena*) and lime (*Tilia*) flowers. Cherries were also renowned in the East for helping to combat mental fatigue, and frequently ten to twenty were taken daily. Oats are also reputed to be one of the best tonics for the nervous system – herbalists will prescribe a tincture of oats to ease frail nerves – and almonds are believed to fortify the nervous system and at the same time to enhance memory and strength. Here is an alternative recipe for almond milk to the one you will find under Measles (see page 114):

Place 2 oz [50 g] of whole almonds in a small saucepan and cover with 7–10 fl oz [200–300 ml] of water. Bring to the boil, and boil for one minute. Remove from the heat, allow to cool, then squeeze the almonds out of their skins. Put the skinned almonds and the water into a liquidiser and blend until smooth.

Anne McIntyre, the Gloucestershire-based herbalist who combines the use of both Western and Eastern herbs, is a great fan of the Ayurvedic herb, ashwagandha (*Withania somnifera*). She says: 'This is a wonder herb. More people have told me their lives have changed due to ashwagandha than any other herb. Nowadays we live on our nerves, we are frazzled and so deplete our energy. Ashwagandha calms you down, grounds you and helps you to conserve the energy we so carelessly fritter away. I strongly recommend it for anyone going through a divorce or coping with too much change. It's a true adaptogen: it changes how you cope with you.'

Here is Anne's recipe for ashwagandha with almond milk:

> Use almond or rue milk, warmed and add a teaspoon of ashwa-gandha powder, a few drops of rosewater, a pinch of cinnamon and jaggery or maple syrup to taste

'This is so self-indulgent. It's like eating Turkish delight, but this will do you nothing but good.'

See also Anxiety; Depression; Insomnia.

Styes

A stye is an infection in the follicle of an eyelash, which becomes a small boil. The most obvious treatment would be to make a small compress to draw the stye to a head, and because styes are so close to the eyes the received wisdom is to use fairly hot water on its own, perhaps with a small amount of salt added or a tiny quantity of pot marigold (*Calendula officinalis*).

However, the remedy that has been most commonly suggested is to rub the affected area gently with a gold ring, preferably a wedding ring. Catherine Gould from Farringdon, Janet Stubbins of Wells and many others recall this tradition, although it has all the signs of being an old wives' tale. The only possible explanation can be that the smooth surface of the ring creates a little warmth as it 'massages' the eye area, so bringing the little boil to a head.

Katherine Cross from Worthing remembers goulard water being used for any eye conditions, including styes. This was bought from a pharmacist, diluted in water and used in an eyebath. In fact, it was made from Goulard's Extract, which was a solution of lead acetate, widely used as an astringent in the nineteenth and early twentieth centuries. It is even mentioned in one of Balzac's stories, where it was used to treat wounds. However, it was a carcinogenic substance and is no longer produced.

Sunburn

My grandmother, Annie Ely Bolton, was a great advocate of bicarbonate of soda. I can remember her applying the paste described below to the shoulders, bald pates, feet and noses of any family member or guest who had inadvertently snoozed in hot sun.

Make a paste from bicarbonate of soda and cool water. Apply the paste directly on to the sunburnt areas or, if the sunburn is extensive, add the bicarbonate of soda in handfuls to a bath of cool water. Sit in this bath for at least 20–30 minutes to take the heat out of the burnt areas. Pat the skin very gently afterwards, but do not rub.

Elaine Brakby from Liverpool also remembers using bicarbonate of soda:

I worked for a large, luxurious hotel on the north Cornish coast in the 1960s and 1970s. If any of our guests were sunburnt, we would give them a packet of bicarbonate of soda. We told them to put it into the bath with the water as cold as they could stand it. It would take the heat out of the burns.

A long-standing traditional remedy is to use elderflower (*Sambucus nigra*) water both for sunburn and to reduce freckles.

Steep the flowers in water or pop them in a muslin bag to steep in bathwater.

A charming and fragrant alternative comes from Jessica Ashley:

Put powdered milk and ten drops of lavender essential oil into a container. Shake it thoroughly and allow it to stand for at least a day. Then pour into bathwater, and enjoy the soak.

Sweaty hands and feet

The French believe in tea to aid sore and smelly feet. Rich in tannins, tea contains drying agents, astringents, and will slow the perspiration that is the main cause of bad odour. A typical French remedy is:

Put two or three teabags into four litres [about 7 pints] of water. Boil for 10 minutes. Allow to cool. Soak the feet for half an hour before drying them carefully.

Much the same remedy pops up in parts of the United States, notably the eastern seaboard and California:

Boil five tea bags for five minutes in a quart [2 pints/1.2 litres] of water. Allow to cool. Soak hands or feet in the liquid for 20–30 minutes.

Teeth cleaning

t The first toothbrush was invented in China and was made from pig bristles – pigs from cold climates were considered the best because their hairs stood erect – inserted into little bamboo handles. Toothbrushes didn't reach Europe until the seventeenth century, when the French were the first to use them. About 2,500 years ago the Chinese also made the first toothpastes. Egyptians, ancient Greeks and Romans also believed in the value of good tooth care and would use a variety of abrasive substances – from burned shells to pumice and powdered flintstone, powdered fruit and talc – as cleaning agents, applied with little twigs or a cloth.

The seventeenth-century herbalist Nicholas Culpeper offers a remedy 'to keep teeth white'. He suggests:

> *Dip a little piece of white cloth in Vinegar of Quinces, and rub your gums with it, for it is of a gallant binding quality, and not only makes the teeth white, but also strengthens the gums, fastens the teeth and also causeth a sweet breath.*

Within living memory, in parts of Ireland soot was a favourite. This was surprisingly effective because it, too, has an abrasive quality. Micheline Walsh from London remembers that her father in Ireland used a mixture of soot and salt (which is antiseptic). She says: 'He had great teeth and kept all of them until he died at the age of seventy-eight.'

Sage (*Salvia*) is such a useful herb, being highly antiseptic, antibacterial and anti-fungal. It's hardly surprising that, among its many medicinal uses, its leaves were often used as a mouth freshener. Culpeper advocated it for 'the rotting and consuming of the gums', and he suggested washing your mouth with sage-water and rubbing a leaf around your mouth. Pamela Jackson from Basingstoke uses it to this day, both to freshen the mouth and to polish her teeth.

Herbalists of the past used to sell liquorice roots that had been cut into sticks. I remember chewing them as a child. Although tasting quite sweet, due to a compound called glycyrrhizin, liquorice counteracts bacteria, and in the seventeenth century it was thought to discourage plague. I also remember being told to use baking soda on the rare occasion we had run out of toothpaste at home. This is a remedy I have often heard so assume it was fairly commonplace.

Cynthia Swift, who now lives in Spain, reminds us that many of our grandmothers – and grandfathers – would use a toothpick. These are still in frequent use in many parts of Europe and are often to be found on restaurant tables, but the habit seems to have died out in Britain. It is still a useful emergency measure to dislodge any particle of food that has become trapped.

See also Halitosis.

Throats (sore)

Soothing is the word that comes to mind when you have a sore throat. Even so, some folk remedies sound fairly abrasive. Norris Winstone from Norwich, who at the time of writing is ninety-four, remembers his London-based grandmother keeping a stick of camphor in a small bottle of brandy to cure a sore throat. He says: 'You drank a few drops of the brandy. Some people said that the sting of the drink was worse than the soreness; others thought it was an excuse to have a drink.'

More soothing for a child is this remedy that Angela Moules, who was a nurse at the Great Ormond Street Hospital for Sick Children in the 1930s, came across. She calls it 'Kogle Mogle':

Beat the yolk of 1 egg with a dessertspoon of caster sugar until the sugar has dissolved.

Anna Davies from London prefers hot milk and garlic, which, of course, is a powerful natural antiseptic.

Heat up half a pint (or quarter of a litre) of milk. Add two cloves of garlic, a teaspoon of butter and some honey to your taste. Drink a whole mug before going to bed.

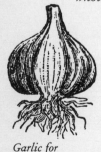

Carola Augustin also believes in garlic but adds that this remedy has a detoxing effect on the body, cleansing every cell. It may cause a strong odour, so this is not a remedy to try before a party or important date.

Knead soft white bread into a ball. Push a clove of garlic into the centre of the ball. Then chew the ball of bread as slowly and for as long as possible.

Garlic for sore throats.

A Hindu remedy comes from Mina Roberts in St Mawgan, Cornwall. In Ayurvedic medicine turmeric has the reputation of having antibiotic properties, which are useful in treating fevers and sore throats.

First warm some milk, and then add a good pinch of saffron and turmeric. You can also add sugar to taste.

There are external remedies for sore throats, too, not least wrapping the throat in a warm scarf or felt overnight. In Austria there is a variation that involves pig's fat:

Put a quantity of pig's fat into a saucepan and put it on a low heat until the fat has melted into a soft spread. Soak a long thin cloth in the softened fat and wrap it around your throat.

However, as a Viennese friend points out, a good cashmere scarf serves the same purpose and looks considerably better.

Gargles are also a traditional part of treatment. Mrs Grieve is among those herbalists who recommend a raspberry leaf tea which is made with an ounce (25 g) of dried raspberry leaves steeped in a pint (600 ml) of boiling water, making a tea that can be used for 'sore mouth and canker of the throat'.

Slightly more worrying, although many people remember this remedy, is the use of permanganate of potash (or potassium permanganate). Dr Vivien Martin of Worthing recalls:

My mother would take five tiny crystals and dissolve them in plenty of water, turning it a marvellous violet colour, to make a gargle.

However, it is worth remembering that potassium permanganate is used as an oxidising agent and disinfectant and in deodorisers and dyes. Beware: it can be poisonous if undiluted and may turn the skin purple.

Finally, writing in the 1870s in her personal book of household hints and medical 'receipts', Kate Fox from Aston, Oxfordshire, advocated:

Eggs can be combined with other ingredients to treat sore throats.

Take the white of 2 eggs and beat them, add 2

teaspoons white sugar, grate in a little nutmeg and then add one pint [600 ml] of lukewarm water. Stir well and drink often.

Ticks

Ticks are little blood-sucking parasites, a little larger than mites, which are their relatives. They sit on tall grass and trees, waiting for a suitable host – dogs, deer and occasionally human beings – to brush by. The tick then attaches itself to the skin with its mouthparts, inserts a probe and draws blood, all with no pain to its host. Often the tick will gorge itself and drop off with no ill effects, but sometimes it will be carrying bacteria that can cause Lyme disease. If the tick is pulled off, leaving the head under the skin, this can also result in infections.

The traditional method of removal is to push down on the skin surrounding the tick and pull carefully away by the head. You can sometimes use tweezers, but they must be used as close to the head as possible. If you hold the tick by its body, it can burst and force contaminants into the skin.

My mother, Joan Chappell, had Scottish terrier dogs, which, being shaped like brooms, were forever picking up ticks. She would tie a length of cotton thread to the tick, as near the head as possible, and slowly pull it out. It is important not to jerk, otherwise the body will come away, leaving the head under the skin.

Tinnitus

A ringing in the ears can be the result of a build-up of wax or of some form of infection or blockage. This may be an indication of an underlying condition, but sometimes the buzzing appears to have no physical reason at all. In traditional Chinese medicine it is believed to be a defence against things people do not wish to hear and is closely related to some form of stress or anxiety.

Some people report relief by massaging the mastoid bone, which lies just behind the ear, using a warm oil. This should be repeated twice a day, morning and late at night. Others find acupuncture of value.

See also Earache.

Toenails

Jim White, a Scot now living in Glendale, California, has fond memories of his grandmother, Janet Robertson, who lived in the small village of Halbeath, near Dunfermline. He recalls her using Vicks vapour rub, a preparation normally used as a rub for the chest, to cure his fungal toenails. He explains:

> *Just coat the toenails with Vicks compound every evening before going to bed. Within a week it usually begins to show that the fungus is dying. Keep applying, and cut the toenails to let the compound soak under the nail. This also softens the nails, making it easier to cut away the nail bit by bit, until the fungus is gone and the new nail has grown in. This takes some time but it does kill the fungus.*

Another remedy is to use distilled vinegar, which contains 5 per cent acetic acid.

Apply to the nail and the cuticle area on a cotton bud first thing in the morning and last thing at night. It is important not to miss an application.

Alternatively, take one part vinegar — white vinegar or even cider apple vinegar — to two parts of lukewarm water and soak the toes for 20 to 30 minutes daily.

Traditional wisdom also suggests that, as with Athlete's foot (see page 9), fermented food and sugar should be avoided in the diet when the body has a fungal infection.

Tonsillitis

Connie Jamieson from Edinburgh recalls that a long, slender brush was used to paint infected tonsils with iodine. As she points out, this method is extremely likely to make the patient retch. Annie Ely Bolton, my grandmother, had two favourite remedies that she would use for sore throats, one using lemons, which have antiseptic qualities, the other using sage.

Mix one to two drops of lemon oil into half a glass of warm milk. Mix and use it as a gargle.

Alternatively,

Chop fresh sage leaves finely and put into a mug. Add salt. Pour in boiling water. Allow the brew to stand until it has cooled. Use as a gargle.

Lemon oil and milk
for sore throats.

Di Spero from north London reports how grateful she was to her friend, Dru Tramaseur from East Sussex, who arrived with the following remedy when Di's throat was so sore that she could hardly speak.

1 tablespoon of natural organic yoghurt
1 clove of garlic, finely chopped
2 pinches of salt

Mix into a paste and keep in the fridge. Take a teaspoon every time you cough. Try to keep the paste at the back of the tongue and let it dissolve gently into the throat.

Di says that this is difficult to achieve, but the cold yoghurt is extremely soothing to a burning throat. However, she did this night and day and her throat quickly improved.

See also Throats (sore).

Toothache

In parts of rural Russia there is a tradition of wedging valerian leaves between aching teeth. Valerian (*Valeriana officinalis*) is sometimes called all-heal, and there is more information about it under Insomnia (see page 107). Dr Henry Oakeley, a Fellow of the Royal College of Physicians, points out that valerian was used as a sedative to the higher nerve centres in conditions of nervous unrest, such as St Vitus's dance, and neuralgic pains. It is just possible, therefore, that localised it may aid toothache.

In 1653 Nicholas Culpeper advised the use of elder (*Sambucus*):

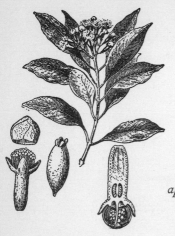

Clove oil for toothache.

Take the inner rind of an Elder-Tree, and bruise it, and put thereto a little Pepper, and make it into balls, and hold them between the teeth that ache.

A Scottish remedy sent in, like so many others from that part of the country, suggests using whisky:

Make a plug of cotton wool, soak it in whisky and apply it to the troublesome tooth.

In *Auld Scottish Grannies' Remedies* by Betty Kirkpatrick there is a saying, 'let the sau sink to the sair', translated literally as 'let the salve sink into the sore place' but more frequently translated as 'drink the whisky rather than just rubbing it in'.

If whisky is not to your liking, there are other widespread remedies, such as putting a pinch of alum or a small piece of clove on the offending tooth, or putting one drop of oil of cloves on to cotton wool and applying this to the gum close to the tooth. If all else fails you could try painting the tooth and surrounding gum with iodine.

To prevent toothache in the first place, it's still recommended to eat apples, which have long been regarded as a good natural dentifrice.

Should the tooth be beyond salvation, removal was the only solution in the past. The earliest dentists were blacksmiths and therefore it is not surprising that some of the equipment that dentists use even today bears a resemblance to a blacksmith's tools.

See also Halitosis; Teeth cleaning.

Travel sickness

There have been reports in learned medical journals about the efficacy of ginger in reducing vomiting and nausea. These findings will come as no surprise to many families (including my own) who have found it the best possible remedy for travel sickness, whether you are travelling by car, coach or boat. You can either use crystallised ginger or take it as a tincture or make a ginger tea before your journey.

> *To make ginger tea: cut a slither of fresh ginger root or use a pinch of dried ginger powder and add to a cup of boiling water. Leave for four to five minutes and then sip. You can add other warming spices, such as cinnamon, if you wish. It's even pleasant drunk cold (but not chilled), so if you are on a long journey, take a little flask with you.*

Tuberculosis

The disease tuberculosis (or TB) was known as consumption in the past because it 'consumed' the body, most particularly the lungs. It has largely been eradicated in the West, although in recent years there has been a worrying trend of recurrence among people whose immune systems are compromised through drug abuse or HIV/AIDS. It is still rampant in many developing countries.

Here is an eighteenth-century remedy for 'lungs water' found in a handwritten book now in the library of the Royal College of Physicians:

Take a gallon [4.5 litres] of milk, the lungs of a calf while warm cut it in pieces, a peck of garden snails washed then beat in a mortar until the snails are broken, 12 whites of eggs, 4 nutmegs in pieces. Distil it in a cold still.

In the instructions, it is also suggested that the results are sweetened with sugar candy or loaf sugar to make it more palatable – I can't help but feel that it would take more than a spoonful of sugar to help this medicine of calf lungs and garden snails go down.

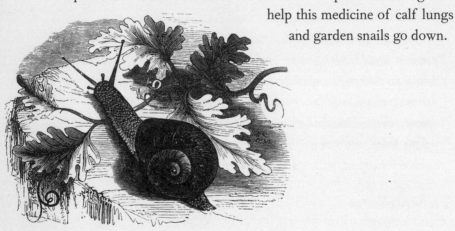

Snails combined with
other ingredients for
tuberculosis.

Ulcers (leg)

Ulcers on the legs, whitlows on fingers and any infected wound may benefit from the application of chickweed (*Stellaria media*). Cynthia Swift's interest in herbs dates from her childhood when she helped an old woman in her village gather the ingredients for her tisanes, creams and poultices – and for elderberry wine. Nowadays, Cynthia lives in Spain, but she has contributed the following remedy:

> *Gather fresh chickweed from clean land and hedgerows. Rinse in cold water to remove any dust or debris. Boil water, pour it over the chickweed and allow it to stand for one minute, then pour away the water. When warm to the touch apply the chickweed directly on to the infected site. Cover with a pad of gauze squares and secure firmly with an elastic bandage and pin. Leave for a minimum of eight hours, preferably overnight. Then, remove the holding bandage and carefully lift off the gauze pad. Burn the dressing and contents immediately.*

Cynthia stresses that it is important not to wash, touch or apply any cream or powder. Repeat the chickweed treatment mornings and evenings. The infection comes away cleanly on to the pad and, after three or four days, new skin begins to grow from the edges to the centre.

In *The Oxford Book of Health Foods* J.G. Vaughan and P.A. Judd acknowledge that chickweed is regarded as having cooling and soothing properties and so has been included in ointments and poultices to treat various skin disorders, including sores and boils, for many centuries. Herbalist Anne McIntyre confirms its use for burns and scalds, ulcers, piles and abscesses. In her book *The Complete Floral Healer* she writes: 'It has drawing properties and helps to bring poisons and pus to the surface.' It can also be added to salads and be cooked as a vegetable.

Sheila Sherrard-Smith, a Scot now living in Surrey, recalls that her father, John MacKenzie, was treated with seaweed poultices for his leg ulcer. The MacKenzie family lived in Tullachard in Perthshire when Sheila was growing up, before she moved to St Andrews. Seaweed would be collected from the beach, wrapped in gauze and bound to John's leg with a bandage and then checked every two days. It was believed that the iodine naturally occurring in the seaweed was beneficial.

Varicose veins

Often painful, varicose veins occur when the flow of blood has become obstructed, and they usually appear in the legs, causing the veins to swell and become 'knotted'. The other area subject to the condition is inside the rectum, resulting in haemorrhoids or piles (see Haemorrhoids). Pregnancy and obesity can be causes, but there may be hereditary causes, too.

My grandmother, Annie Ely Bolton, wore heavy, tight stockings to relieve the ache of her varicose veins, particularly when she was likely to be standing for any length of time. She also drank tea made from butcher's broom (*Ruscus aculeatus*). It has been confirmed by German researchers that butcher's broom decreases the inflammation of the veins and helps to strengthen them.

Another herbal remedy to be taken internally for reducing inflammation is St John's wort (*Hypericum perforatum*), and this has value when it is used externally in the form of a salve or an ointment.

Relief may also be gained from compresses applied to affected areas. Native Americans used witch hazel (*Hamamelis* spp.), trees found throughout North America. Rich in tannins, flavonoids and essential oils, witch hazel not only has astringent properties but also, trials show, can check bleeding. Another herb that is naturalised in North America, yarrow (*Achillea millefolium*), has similar properties and a long history of use for wounds and inflammations.

St John's wort for varicose veins.

The French also believe in the value of compresses for engorged and painful veins. Many a *grandmère* would recommend:

> *Mixing together one litre [1¾ pints] of olive oil, two cups of cider vinegar and a large glass of lukewarm water. Soak a length of fine cotton in the mixture and apply to the painful parts for twenty minutes. Refresh the compress when necessary.*

Verrucas and warts

There is something rather curious about our attitude to warts. Maybe it is because over the ages they have come to represent blemishes of devilish interest – or at the very least a sign of extreme ugliness. Ask a child or a horror film designer to create a witch or a crone, and the chances are that they will cover the face with large and nasty warts.

In fact, warts – and verrucas, which are the painful form that grow on the soles of the feet – are caused by a virus. Orthodox medicine suggests there are two methods of treatment: a 'paint' of salicylic acid or applications of liquid nitrogen to burn them away.

However, unlike most other conditions, people ascribe mystical properties to these little growths and subscribe to strange remedies to cure them. There were even claims that certain gifted people could 'charm' the warts away. Margaret Lynas of Lisnaskea in Northern Ireland knew of children who had been taken to a person who would charm the wart by rubbing it round and round with his thumb. The wart would allegedly disappear within days but, Margaret adds, no money was allowed to change hands or the charm would not work. Marguerite Hughes from Birmingham remembers a large, well-known and respected chemist shop called Galloways in the centre of the city that offered to charm warts away. People would place their names in a book in the shop and wait for their warts to disappear. There's no record of the success rate.

Another magical remedy I have come across a number of times is rubbing the wart with a small piece of raw meat, which is then buried in the ground. As the meat rots, expect your wart to disappear. People have averred in all honesty that it worked for them.

Less unlikely but still requiring a leap of faith, Richard Harry, a retired blacksmith and farrier from St Nicholas in south Wales, recalls having groups of gypsy men and women calling at his forge to collect 'bosh' or 'bosch' water in bottles for use in treating warts. This was the water into which hot iron had been plunged to temper it. Richard and his wife were so fascinated by this remedy that they tried it themselves and believe it to have worked.

Annie Penfold (see page 209) has a more practical remedy.

Tie a single horsehair around a wart. Pull it tight and leave it in place until the wart drops off.

Annie's daughter, Angelina, had three warts on her cheek and used this method. It worked and she has no scarring. Cyril Law from County Down also subscribes to this method, as does Connie Jamieson from Edinburgh, although she advocates using a cotton thread instead of the horsehair.

Several people recommend using the white sap from a dandelion (*Taraxacum officinale*). Both Norris Winstone from Norfolk and Jennifer Harper Deacon in her 'What's the Alternative' column in the *Sunday Times* Style magazine recall it. So does Dot Alsworth from Witney in Oxfordshire. She was raised in Lancashire and developed a lot of warts on her knees. Her grandmother, Julia Fenney from Widnes, used this remedy, which Dot insists worked, although she says it took a few weeks.

The method is to squeeze out the milky sap that oozes from the base of the leaf or stalk of a dandelion, and apply it to the site of the wart. Use it twice a day.

Carol Miller, a reflexologist from Lanivet, Cornwall, strongly recommends using radishes. Take the end off a fresh radish and cut a thin slice. Rub the slice over the verruca for a few seconds and then throw it away. Repeat regularly – a bunch of radishes lasts for ages – and continue until the verruca disappears. Carol adds: 'My friend, Rosemarie tried it on a verruca and it worked brilliantly, so I tried it on a small wart and it worked for that too.'

Other people have suggested applying oil of lemon to a wart twice a day, while others opt for rubbing the under skin of a banana, again twice a day, on to the wart. There's even some support for potato water (the water in which potatoes have been boiled), which should be used as a lotion to treat warts. Last but not least, Jean Rogerson from Bolton opts for using a match head. She explains that you should wet the end of an unstruck match and rub it on to the wart. The sulphur in the match head seems to be the magic ingredient here.

Vomiting

In *A Modern Herbal* (1931) Mrs Grieve espoused the use of dandelion (*Taraxacum officinale*), writing: 'When the stomach is irritated and where active treatment would be injurious, the decoction or extract of Dandelion administered three or four times a day, will often form a valuable remedy.'

Her recipe for dandelion tea was to infuse one ounce (15 g) of dandelion in a pint (600 ml) of boiling water for 10 minutes. This was then decanted and sweetened with honey. Patients would then drink several glasses in the course of a day. Mrs Grieve stated: 'The use of this tea is efficacious in bilious affections.' This is a similar remedy to that mentioned as a liver tonic on page 111.

Dandelion extract for an upset stomach.

Wasp stings

W

There seems to be one sovereign remedy for wasp stings, and it crops up all over the country. It is quite simply vinegar, which should be applied liberally to the site, once the sting has been removed. Another lesser-known remedy was to make a paste of vinegar with baking soda.

Within living memory in this country and in the United States, people would apply chewed tobacco to the site of a sting. Needless to say, now that the hazards of tobacco are well known, this practice has died out.

Whooping cough

In these days of antibiotics, whooping cough (pertussis), nasty as it is, can easily be treated. In former times, however, it was an extremely serious condition, and there are many remedies that purported to alleviate the symptoms. Barbara Sanginson from Ripon in north Yorkshire remembers being treated by a remedy using wild garlic when she was a child over seventy years ago.

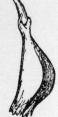

Protecting the skin with one or two layers of socks, apply slices of wild garlic root to the soles of the feet, keeping them in place with another layer of socks. Caution: if the garlic touches the skin it will cause severe blisters. The patient's breath will soon smell very strongly of garlic.

Garlic for whooping cough.

Barbara says: 'This was my grandmother's remedy and used by my mother when I had whooping cough. We had plenty of wild garlic growing nearby, but the cultivated type would presumably be just as effective.'

Another remedy originates in Lincolnshire. Pauline Clayton from Barnetby recalls being a victim of a raging whooping cough epidemic more than fifty years ago, and her mother, Dorothy Broddle, used a remedy she had learned from her great-aunt, Susan Gilliat.

¼ pint [150 ml] white vinegar
1 egg
1 lb [500 g] white sugar
red lavender liquid (about 1½ fl oz/38 ml)

The red lavender liquid (presumably a tincture) was available from the chemist. Certainly Pauline remembers that 'the taste was not unpleasant and it took the "whoop" out of the cough.'

It is a remedy not unlike the one Sheila Sherrard-Smith was given in her childhood in Scotland, which used three parts of honey to one of white vinegar. It was left in a saucer by her bed at night, to be taken with a teaspoon. Sheila says that she used the preparation for her children, and they use it now for theirs.

In her book of handwritten remedies dating from the 1860s or 1870s, Kate Fox from Aston in Oxfordshire records:

1 scruple Salts of Tartar dissolved in ¼ pint [150 ml] cold water, add 10 grains cochineal finely powdered and sweeten with loaf sugar very sweet. Give to an Infant a teaspoonful 4 times a day, a child 3 years old ½ tablespoonful. According to age increase quantity.

To be rubbed in chest for same: ¼ lb [125g] lard, 2 oz [50g] camphor to be simmered together and well rubbed in night and morning.'

Kate makes a note that this remedy was given to her by Mrs Selfe. Meanwhile, a Mr Patterson gave her another remedy for a rub for whooping cough:

> *Pour ¼ pt rum [150 ml] on 2d (two pennyworth) Garlic (cut up fine, let it stand) rub well into the Chest and Back.*

Mrs Grieve, however, in *A Modern Herbal* (1931), states firmly of the herb thyme: 'The pounded herb, if given fresh, from 1 oz to 6 oz [25–175 g] daily, mixed with syrup, has been employed with success as a safe cure for whooping cough.' She also gives a recipe for an infusion of thyme. One ounce (25 g) of dried thyme is used to one pint (600 ml) of boiling water, sweetened with sugar or honey, is given for whooping cough, but she suggests it is equally effective in cases of catarrh and sore throat. She suggests giving doses of one or more tablespoonsful, several times daily and adds that 'the wild plant may be equally well used for this'.

Worms

Many small children experience threadworms, and both children and adults can pick up tapeworms from contaminated food. Tapeworms, in particular, can be difficult to get rid of. For centuries herbalists and naturopaths have prescribed a fast of at least twelve hours, followed by a remedy that uses pumpkin seeds and castor oil:

> *Take 2 oz [50 g] of fresh pumpkin seeds. Dip them into very hot water so you can easily remove the skins. Place the seeds in a pestle or basin and mash them, adding a few drops of milk to produce a paste. Take the mixture at the end of the fast. Two hours later, take*

four teaspoons of castor oil (you can add fruit juice to make it palatable). The tapeworm should be passed within three to four hours.

A variation of this treatment is, as before, to refrain from eating any food, then:

Take 1½ oz [40 g] of fresh pumpkin seeds and 2 cloves of garlic, mash to a pulp and split the mixture into three portions. Take one portion for breakfast, one for lunch and the third for supper. Take a herbal laxative before bedtime. Children from 2 to 5 should only take one-third of the dose and children from 6 to 10 only half.

Saints, Witches and Wise Women
Women and Medicine Throughout History

When I was gathering the material for this book I became intrigued by the way that throughout history women seem to have been marginalised from the medical professions while occupying a central role in everyday family healthcare. Indeed, for many centuries women in the West were forbidden to become doctors, leading to a gender inequality in the health services that is only today beginning to be rectified. If we look further back into history, however, there is some evidence of women who were regarded as healers in much the same way as men were. Australian Aboriginal women were the healers of their tribes, with traditional knowledge and philosophy being passed down verbally from generation to generation. Now that their culture has been all but destroyed, this wealth of knowledge has almost vanished, though thankfully some Australian universities are gathering and recording what is left.

In ancient Somalia and Egypt women were priestesses as well as healers, and they were honoured and considered powerful in their societies. The Egyptian goddess Isis promoted healing and the dispensing of healing herbs. Several of the queens of Egypt, including Hatshepsut (c.1540–c.1481 BC), encouraged women to study medicine. Anaesthesia and surgery were advanced, and, of course, we are acquainted with their deep understanding of anatomy and the extent of their skills through the embalming and preservation of the dead. Records show that there were schools of medicine, and some of the papyrus accounts of remedies and treatments have survived. We also know that there were extensive medicinal herb gardens, and there is a well-known depiction in a physician's tomb that dates back about 5,000 years of patients receiving reflexology treatments.

There were women physicians, some of whom are well documented, in both Greek times and in ancient Rome. It was the decline of the Roman Empire and the onset of the Dark Ages that resulted in a tragic loss of knowledge and a downturn in medical practice.

The Early Church

The early Church set about eradicating all pre-Christian culture, including the knowledge and wisdom in science and medicine that had accumulated over thousands of years. There was even a ban on the study of medicine. In its place came the doctrines of superstition: that all diseases were caused by sinful behaviour and by evil spirits for which the only treatment was exorcism. These were truly the Dark Ages.

Individual women found it increasingly difficult to retain their place as healers, but exceptions were to be found in monasteries and the convents. It was to these centres that the needy, sick and disabled flocked, and monks and nuns would do what they could to alleviate the suffering. Eventually, during the Middle Ages, more enlightened rulers – or their wives – established hospitals and schools of medicine in these religious centres. Eleanor of Aquitaine (1122–1204), for instance, and her daughters and granddaughters after her, established hospitals, clinics, pharmacies and also sanctuaries for lepers.

Wars took a toll, but even wholesale slaughter took second place to the terrible impact of plague. The Black Death, when it took hold in the mid-fourteenth century, is believed to have caused the deaths of between one-third and half the population of Europe. Societies and communities were, literally, decimated. Plague reappeared on a regular basis and so continued to be feared throughout the Tudor and Stuart periods.

Witchcraft and Wise Women

Women faced other challenges as healers. The early Church taught women that their normal bodily processes were sinful and 'unclean'. Women were meant to bear the discomfort of menstruation and the pain of childbirth without complaint because these were seen as punishment for the 'Sin of Eve'. Trotula di Ruggerio (see pages 178–80) did not believe this, and nor, a century or so later, did the equally gifted healer, Hildegard of Bingen (see pages 182–86).

If they became prominent or showed talent women healers also risked the accusation of using 'magic' and were therefore subject to the charge of witchcraft. This was a dreadful period, when thousands of women were subjected to appalling torture and death on the basis of spiteful and unjust accusations. In her book *Women Healers Through History* Elisabeth Brooke quotes the tragic example of Alison Peirson of Byrehill in Scotland who had established a reputation as a gifted – if rather fey – healer: 'The Archbishop of St Andrews was suffering from an illness which the orthodox physicians could not heal. He sent for Alison and she healed him. After he was better, the archbishop declared she was a witch, refused to pay her for her work.' Not only was poor Alison arrested and tried for 'using magical powers', but in May 1588 she was burned at the stake for witchcraft. One can only hope that the ungrateful archbishop's sickness recurred.

Elisabeth Brooke writes:

> *I believe that the Inquisition was a carefully and cynically planned and executed assault on women who dared to move out of the narrow limits set down for them, especially in the field of medicine where women were able to express their humanitarian tendencies. Men were afraid of the power and influence that women possessed and also of their possible rebellion against the patriarchal status quo. If women remained submissive, passive and uneducated they were left alone, but those few who managed to educate themselves and set themselves up as authorities in their given subjects, and particularly those within the medical profession, had to be destroyed. Their intuitive and scientific knowledge meant that they posited a real threat to inadequate and greedy male physicians.*

Moving On

Healthcare in the seventeenth, eighteenth and early nineteenth centuries continued to be of low standard. Infant mortality was high, despite efforts to establish good practice in midwifery. The great herbalist Nicholas Culpeper wrote a widely distributed book for midwives, and Mrs Elizabeth Cellier tried to establish midwifery as a profession with study and standard working practices. Even though she was granted a Royal Charter in 1687, her valiant efforts came to nothing.

In the North American colonies, however, women were free to study and practise, and they were soon becoming accomplished midwives, doctors and nurses. We know a little about the herbs that the Pilgrim Fathers (and Mothers) took with them, and undoubtedly they also learned from Native American healers.

In Britain – and indeed throughout western Europe – herbal medicine was in decline during the 1800s. As the Royal College of Physicians points out, their place in the home medicine chest was taken by noxious chemical preparations, including laudanum, opium and calomel (mercury). Quietly, however, botanical societies continued to exist, and in Britain in 1846 a number of practitioners came together to found the National Association of Medical Herbalists 'to encourage the study and knowledge of the vegetable kingdom and its application to public health'.

Despite their work, it was not until 1927 that Hilda Leyel opened the Culpeper shops, founded the Herb Society and formed her famous association with Mrs Maud Grieve.

In orthodox medicine it was only in the late nineteenth century that women made real progress, and it was the early twentieth century before they were allowed to enter the orthodox medical schools and to qualify and practise. The battle continued throughout much of the last century as women gradually gained footholds not only in every medical specialty but at all levels. The first woman to be elected president of the Royal College of Physicians was Dame Margaret Turner Warwick in 1989.

Throughout the centuries there were many heroines, and the pages that follow offer potted biographies of just a few of them. From Trotula to Mary Seacole, they represent the women who quietly and determinedly ignored the politics and continued their quest to understand how the human body works and to discover what could be done to maintain it or cure it when it fails to function. We salute them all.

Saint of Herbs — *Anastasia*

In Byzantine art you will find icons of St Anastasia holding bottles of medicine and herbs. In Greece she is known as *pharmakolytra*, meaning the one who saved people with medicine. The details of her life remain tantalisingly hazy, and much is no more than supposition. However, one persistent legend has it that she visited the prisons where Christians were being held and tortured in order to treat their wounds.

Although there is little substantive fact, it is believed that she was born in Rome of a noble family, possibly the daughter of Praetextus, and was introduced to Christianity by her mother. Some sources suggest that she married a pagan, Publius, who ill-treated her when he discovered her strong Christian faith. It is said that she was a spiritual student of St Chrysogonus, who was martyred in the time of the emperor Diocletian in the year 303. There are several versions of Anastasia's death, which was possibly in the following year, 304. Some reports suggest that she was beheaded, others that she was burned, but most suggest that she was executed at Sirmium in Dalmatia (Sremska Mitrovica, Serbia), also a victim of Diocletian's persecutions. There is even confusion about where her remains lie. She was first buried in the cathedral at Zadar, Croatia, but her relics may have later been transferred to the Cathedral of Anastasia in Istanbul.

What is clear is that she has been revered as a healer and doctor-saint for many centuries. Her name is commemorated in the Roman Catholic Church, and her feast day is 25 December, Christmas Day.

The Greek Orthodox Church honours her on 22 December, and even today, in some areas of northern Greece, special bread with herbs is made on her feast day, and people place herbs on her icon.

The Mother of Gynaecology
— Trotula di Ruggerio

Throughout the Middle Ages Salerno was the greatest and most influential of the European centres of natural medicine. Located not far from Naples on the coast of southern Italy, it was not only a seat of learning but its hospitals also had a worldwide reputation for excellence.

From at least the ninth century onwards, Salerno drew the sick and those wounded during the Crusades, as well as students and teachers who wished to study medicine. The first non-religious school was based there, and legend has it that it was created by four masters: a Greek, a Jew, an Arab and a Latin. Certainly it attracted scholars and physicians from every faith. It is also possible that the school was heavily influenced by Arabic medicine.

For one period in its history women were allowed to study and practise there, and the greatest of them all was Trotula di Ruggerio, who became known throughout the world simply as Trotula. Little is known about her life. She lived at some time in the eleventh century, and some sources believe that she came from a wealthy family. Other sources suggest that she was married and had children and that she held a chair of medicine at the school. What is clear is that she was a pioneer in the treatment of women's conditions and diseases. Her areas of specialty were obstetrics, gynaecology, skin disease and cosmetics. Her work remained a leading authority on women's health for many centuries to come.

She wrote two works, the *Passionibus Mulierum Curandorum* (The Diseases of Women), which is known as the Trotula Major, and a second book, known as the Trotula Minor. The authorship of these books has been challenged many times, and this is undoubtedly because she wrote in a very frank, if not explicit, way about female anatomy and sexuality. Women patients no doubt found it easier to discuss intimate matters with her rather than with a male doctor.

Some of her thinking was radical and went against the current beliefs of the Church. For instance, she did not believe that women should suffer the pain of childbirth without relief, as punishment for the Sin of Eve. Instead, she advocated the use of opiates. She also held that a failure to conceive might be the result of a defect in the man as much as the woman. As a consequence, although her texts and work were the basis of treatment for centuries afterwards, some historians and authorities refused even to believe in her existence. Others, hostile to the concept that women could be intellectuals, pioneers and healers, assumed and perpetuated the belief that she must have been a man. This was despite a number of contemporary references to her greatness. She is even mentioned in *The Canterbury Tales* (late 1380s), where she is referred to as Dame Trot.

In the Trotula Major she aimed to educate male doctors about the female body. At that time, as for many centuries later, men were not allowed to examine a female patient intimately and were not present at childbirth. Their knowledge of female anatomy was therefore limited. In her work of sixty-three chapters, she advises women about menstruation, conception, pregnancy, Caesarean sections, childbirth and post-partum care. She also promoted paediatrics as a separate branch of medicine.

In addition, Trotula gave a great deal of general medical advice. She believed, for example, that there were three different kinds of diseases – inherited, contagious and self-generated – and she stressed the need for accurate observation and questioning of patients:

> When you reach the patient, ask where his pain is. Then feel his pulse, touch his skin to see if he has a fever, as if he has had a chill, and when the pain began and if it is worse at night. Watch his facial expression, test the softness of his abdomen and ask if he passes urine frequently, look carefully at the urine, examine his body for sensitive spots and if you find nothing, ask what other doctors he has consulted and what was their diagnosis, ask if he has ever had a similar attack and when. Then having found the cause of his trouble it will be easy to determine his treatment.

She also urged that patients should be treated gently, recommending warm herbal baths, special diets, scented oils for massage, herbal steam infusions and periods of long convalescence.

The Wisdom of the Lady of the Lake
— The Physicians of Myddfai

There is a charming legend in Carmarthenshire about a Lady of the Lake. A young man tending his cattle saw her and, struck with love by her beauty, offered her bread and cheese. She refused his offer, but he tried again on several more occasions, and finally she agreed to marry him. They were married on the condition that if he struck her three times their marriage contract would be broken and she would return to the lake. It was a happy marriage, and the couple had three sons. One day on the way to a christening, her husband struck her jokingly with a pair of gloves: the first blow. On another day, at a wedding, he accidentally tapped her shoulder: the second blow. Finally, he tapped her again at a funeral. As foretold, she left him and returned to the lake, leaving her family heartbroken.

The Lady of the Lake had educated her eldest son, Rhiwallon Feddyg, in medicine and healing, using the many herbs that grew in profusion in the area. She predicted that he would become a great physician, and his family would after him. His sons, Cadwygan, Gruffudd and Einion, became doctors to Rhys Gryg, the lord of Dinefwr in the thirteenth century. From then on, until the eighteenth century, the family continued to practise medicine, setting down a tradition of healthcare that has resonance today. Their achievements are celebrated in a special permanent exhibition at the National Botanic Garden of Wales at Llanarthne in Carmarthenshire.

The manuscripts of the physicians of Myddfai, now in the British Museum and in Oxford, give instructions for diagnosis and treatment, including surgery, the letting of blood and cauterisation, all of which were then common practices. More fascinating – and what brought them international acclaim – was their knowledge of herbs. They left lists of remedies and instructions on how to maintain health, and they placed great importance on good hygiene, healthy eating and exercise.

A Visionary Healer
– Hildegard of Bingen

Born into a wealthy and noble family in Böckelheim, Germany, in 1098, Hildegard became one of the most extraordinary women of her time. She was renowned as a mystic, saint, poet, theologian, intellectual, musician and, at a time when few women could write, the author of many books on spirituality, divinity and natural medicine.

By her own account, she had her first vision before she was five years old. When she was eight her parents sent her to a strict Benedictine order at the convent of Disibodenberg (Diessenberg), where she was enclosed within the cell of an anchoress, Jutta. To be an anchorite meant being walled-up for life, with food passed into the cell and waste passed out. In some instances, although clearly not at Disibodenberg, the doors were blocked. However, in the years that followed, the order grew substantially and became an open order, and it was into this less reclusive life that Hildegard took the veil as a Benedictine nun when she was fifteen.

This was a period in which women could not study at university. Hildegard's initial education was undertaken by Jutta, who taught her to read and to recite the Psalter. The daughter of Count Stephen of Spanheim, Jutta, reputedly a beautiful woman, had rejected marriage and chosen the life of an anchoress. Her reputation for piety drew many young women of good birth to her cell, but she seems to have taken a special interest in Hildegard and arranged for her to have a tutor. This was a monk called Volmar, and it was to him that Hildegard confided her concerns and confusion about her increasingly vivid visions. Over a thirty-year period until his death he was to became both Hildegard's secretary and her friend.

It is more than probable that as part of her duties Hildegard was actively involved in some form of medical practice. This may have been both for those within the convent and also for outsiders who came seeking cures. This would explain her knowledge of obstetrics and gynaecology. It is unlikely that she would have gained her acquaintance of sexual conduct and childbirth within the cloister walls in any other way.

In 1136 Jutta died, and Hildegard succeeded her as abbess. Encouraged by Volmar, she wrote in some detail about her visions and prophesies in a book she called *Scivias* (1141–52), and it was this work that brought her to the attention of the ecclesiastical authorities, including Pope Alexander III.

By 1150, following a vision, she moved with twenty nuns to Rupertsberg, near Bingen, and the community was later granted its own charter. The move came about despite considerable opposition, both at the loss of revenue from the 'dowries' of the twenty nuns and also of the attention and 'gifts' that Hildegard now commanded. It was at Rupertsberg that she wrote her medicinal doctrines, *Physica* (Natural History) and *Causae et curae* (Causes and Cures). As with Trotula, Hildegard's authorship of these two books has been questioned, perhaps because it was assumed that no woman could understand so much about the human body and human behaviour. Others have no doubt of Hildegard's authorship.

Physica is an encyclopaedia of natural history, covering the elements, plants, trees, jewels and stones, metals, fish, birds, animals and reptiles. The section on plants and herbs is particularly interesting. Hildegard believed that the balance or lack of balance of the humours – hot, cold, dry or damp – determined good or poor health. She ascribed the humoral quality to each type of plant and sometimes included a description of its medical uses. For example, a 'cold' plant would be useful against fever. It is not possible to know if she was reflecting the common wisdom of the day or whether she was writing from her own experiences. Certainly, the principle of the humours was widely held in the twelfth century, although Hildegard had her own variations on this theme. She stressed the need for a simple, balanced diet, lack of stress and rest and relaxation.

In one of the sections of *Causae et curae* Hildegard addressed human sexuality, and there is a substantial discussion of the differences between men and women. She subscribed to the belief that sexual intercourse should take place only between married couples for the purposes of procreation – the party line of the Church in that period – and she offered a number of views about the best times for conception to occur. However, while she suggested that women are not more lustful than men (as common opinion held at the time), she wrote openly of the passionate experience of women. Here is her famous description of lovemaking from a woman's point of view:

> When a woman is making love with a man, a sense of heat in her brain, which brings with it sensual delight, communicates the taste of that delight during the act and summons forth the emission of the man's seed. And when the seed has fallen into its place, that vehement heat descending from her brain draws the seed to itself and holds it, and soon the woman's sexual organs contract, and all the parts that are ready to open up during the time of menstruation now close, in the same way as a strong man would hold something enclosed in his fist.

At the same time, Hildegard believed that most women would prefer to remain celibate where they had a choice. Although she avoided the issues of contraception and abortion – both strongly opposed by the Church – she gave several remedies that might trigger an abortion. She also believed, as Trotula did, that a failure to conceive could be either a male or female deficiency. Some of her conclusions are wide of the mark – she believed, for example, that the strength of a man's seed would decide the sex of the child (strong seed making a boy child, weak seed producing a girl).

Other sections of *Causae et curae* are wholly practical, suggesting herbal remedies – some of which appear in the *Physica* – along with recommendations for massage, special diets, herbal infusions, hot baths and rest. She listed various medical conditions, from migraine – from which Hildegard herself is believed to have suffered – to urinary incontinence and worms, each with its remedy. In her book *Hildegard of Bingen: A Visionary Life* Sabina Flanagan says:

> *There is little doubt that the material bears Hildegard's own stamp, although it is hard to conceive of the original form of medicinal and scientific work ... The attention paid to women and the sexual dimension of life also sets Hildegard's work apart from other medieval writings with which it might be compared.*

To the Manor Born
– Lady Margaret Hoby

In the sixteenth and early seventeenth centuries physicians still held on to the medieval belief that four 'humours' made up the human constitution: blood, phlegm, yellow bile and black bile. Illness was caused by an imbalance of these humours and could be righted by diet, purgatives or blood-letting. Surgery was crude and undertaken without anaesthetic, and barbers also practised as surgeons, first shaving people and then letting their blood. The red and white pole traditionally displayed outside barbers' shops is a hangover from this dual role.

The blights of the day included tuberculosis, dysentery (the blood flux) and ague, which was, in fact, a mild but persistent form of malaria. And there were two great fears: sweating sickness and the plague or Black Death. There were no treatments for either, other than fleeing from the sites of outbreak. Sufferers faced a lonely death.

In Tudor times, as before and afterwards, medical schools and formal medical training were not accessible to women. Despite this, family and community health was largely the domain of women, who would rely on age-old practices and their own experience. Where there was a large estate it was often the lady of the manor who took responsibility for the midwifery and the general health not only of her own family but also of all the servants, estate workers and their families.

Elizabeth, Countess of Shrewsbury, better known as Bess of Hardwick, was one such. Another was Lady Margaret Hoby, who is famed for keeping an extraordinary diary – rare amongst Elizabethan women – of her daily and spiritual activities. Born in Linton, Yorkshire, in c.1570–71, Lady Margaret was married three times. An heiress in her own right, when she was seventeen years old she married into a very prominent family – her first husband was Walter Devereux, the younger brother of Robert, Earl of Essex, a favourite of Elizabeth I. The Hackness estate near Scarborough in the North Riding of Yorkshire was acquired for the young couple, but sadly, after two years of marriage, Walter was killed in Rouen, when an armed force, headed by his older brother, was sent to support Henry IV, King of France, against the French Catholics.

Margaret's second marriage was to Thomas Sidney, whom she had known from childhood. He came from an even more illustrious and wealthy family, and his mother was a lady-in-waiting to the queen. This marriage was also short lived, and Margaret became a widow for a second time. She was devastated by Thomas's death – it was rumoured to have been a true love match – and she initially rejected the approaches made to her by Sir Thomas Posthumous Hoby. He persisted and eventually Margaret agreed to marry him.

It was after her marriage to Hoby and while she was living at Hackness, that she started her diary, initially as an account of her spiritual affairs. Margaret was a fervent Puritan and exceptionally devout, and her life revolved around her daily prayers, both public and private, meditation, self-examination and attendance at church. The diary also contains details of her life, which was spent organising and administering the estate and lands around it and caring for her servants, workmen and tenants. The estate was largely self-sufficient, with the gardens providing a range of produce, a proportion duly preserved for winter. There was a granary and bakery and stretches of water stocked with fish. Bees were kept, for honey and, presumably, for beeswax; Margaret records in her diary the occasions when she made wax candles. As part of her 'huswiffrie' (housewifery), her diary also documents the making of preserves and sweetmeats, 'stilling' (possibly ale or a fermented grain), tending her bees, spinning wool, dyeing cloth, gardening, sewing and embroidering, and fishing. In addition, she maintained the estate accounts, intervened in local disputes and kept up a stream of personal correspondence. She also entertained guests on occasion and oversaw the training of young people who were lodged for that purpose in her household.

All these duties were performed despite her own recurring bouts of poor health. She frequently took to her bed and sometimes required the attendance of her appointed physician. There are references to her 'febelnis of stomak and paine of my head' (feebleness of stomach and pain of my head), and she notes taking 'medesone' or 'phesicke' (medicine or physic) and of how she was 'lett blood' (blood-letting). Some sources suggest that she suffered from rheumatism or weakness caused by a deficient diet, but this cannot be verified. Whatever her debility, it might account for the fact that, in three marriages, she did not have any children. Poor Lady Margaret was also plagued by toothache.

Throughout her diary we know that she took seriously her responsibilities for the health of her staff. She mentions reading a herbal, and there are references to growing herbs in her garden. One of the leading herbals of the time was by John Gerard, *The Herball, or Generall Historie of Plantes* (1597), and it had illustrations of each plant, together with its medicinal properties.

Margaret attended childbirths both among her own family, twice for her cousin Ison's wife, and among families on the estate, and she regularly visited the sick and dying. She also spent time talking to the housebound old women, the 'good wives' as she calls them. Domestic injuries were common. On one occasion she dressed a deep cut on the hand of a servant, Jarden, and the following day attended to a 'poore boyes legge that was hurt'. The notes over the following weeks shows that she applied daily dressings to her patients. In July 1600 she records making a 'purgatione', some form of purgative to cleanse the body, for 'my Cosine Isons woman'. A few months later she mentions that she gave a salve or ointment to a 'poore woman of Caton' for her arm.

One entry simply says that 'Blakeborn cutt his foot with a hatchet'. And she then tends this wound – the entries reading, 'dressed Blackbourn's legge' – for the following week. Within a few days another servant, Packering, required his hand to be treated. Lady

Margaret's skill must have been widely known because in 1601 she tells of how a child was brought to her who 'had no fundement, and had no passage for excrementes but att the Mouth'. She was asked to 'cutt the place to se if any passhage Could be made'. She 'cutt deepe and searched [but] there was none to be found'. On another occasion she visited 'Munkmans wife who was sore aflicted in minde'.

One illness for which there was no cure was the plague, and the only 'remedy' was to move away from any area of infection. Lady Margaret was with her husband in London for the funeral of Elizabeth I in April 1603, and within weeks the new king, James I, issued a proclamation that everyone should leave the city because of an outbreak of plague and not return until his coronation. The Hobys quickly returned home, and on 28 June Lady Margaret noted: 'We Came safe, I praise god, to Hacknis' (Harkness). Within weeks, news of the spread of the disease reached them: in one week 3,200 people had died in London – the total was to be ten times that number – and cases were found in the north too, in nearby Hull and Whitby. There were further cases for many months to come.

Unfortunately, we don't have a record of the actual remedies used by Lady Margaret Hoby, but we can piece together some ideas. At one point in her diaries she refers to gathering apples. In the sixteenth century apples were often served at the end of meals, and some varieties were used to make cider. They were also regarded as a remedy for constipation. According to John Gerard, apple pulp mixed with swine's grease and rosewater was made into an ointment. She also preserved quinces that, according to another great herbalist, Nicholas Culpeper, would help 'all sort of fluxes in men or women'. With the addition of vinegar, quince would 'stir up the languishing appetite', and, with honey, would become a purge. Rhubarb was added to deal with phlegm.

Lady Margaret may also have used distilled water of roses. As in the Ayurvedic tradition, rosewater was regarded as good for the heart and for pain in the eyes. She might have made 'pastilles', which were burned to sweeten the air in sickrooms, and she would have been responsible for keeping a supply of the most commonly used herbs.

Advice to Tudor Housewives
— Thomas Tusser

Much of what we know about Elizabethan remedies is derived from an unsuccessful East Anglian farmer named Thomas Tusser (c.1524–80). Thomas came from Essex and possessed a beautiful voice. He became a chorister at the chapel at Wallingford Castle in Berkshire and later at St Paul's. He was sent to Eton, which he loathed, and then went up to Trinity Hall, Cambridge. Later he was appointed musician to his first patron, Lord Paget. He married and moved to Suffolk to farm. This was a dreadful period in his life, for the farm failed and his wife died. He subsequently married a Norfolk girl who gave him four children. He found a further patron in John of Salisbury, dean of Norwich Cathedral, who employed him to oversee cathedral music and the choir, and Thomas's attempts at farming – all disastrous – continued. He died in a debtor's jail in London.

Before then, however, Thomas wrote a calendar of a farmer's year in verse which became a bestseller in Tudor times and has rarely been out of print since. The first edition was *A Hundredth Goode Pointes of Husbandrie*, and it was published in 1557, but after his marriage Tusser added a similar number of points on 'huswifry'. By 1573 the number had increased again, and it was published as *Five Hundred Points of Good Husbandry*. Sadly, he never benefited from his book's success.

Under 'Necessarie Herbes to Growe in a Garden for Physick' (like all written English of the time, the spellings were frequently phonetic), he lists: 'annis, archangel, betanie, charviel, gragons, detaunie (or garden ginger), gromel seed for the stone, hartsong, horehound, lovage for the stone, licoras, mandrake, mogwort, pionees, popie, rew, rubarb, smalach for swellings, saxefrage for the stone, stitchwort, valarian, woodbine'.

Thomas also added a few verses on 'physicke' to guide housewives who read his lines:

> Good huswives provide, ere an sicknes doo come,
> Of sundrie good things in hir house to have some.
> Good Aqua composita, Vineger tart,
> Rosewater and treacle, to comfort the hart.

> Cold herbes in hir garden for agues that burne,
> That over strong heat to good temper may turne,
> While Endive and Suckerie, with Spinnage ynough,
> All such with good pot herbes should follow the plough.

> *Get water of Fumentorie, Liver to coole,*
> *And others the like, or els lie like a foole.*
> *Conserve of the Barberie, Quinces and such,*
> *With Sirops that easeth the sickly so much.*

He also recommends a good diet and relaxation:

> *Good broth and good keeping doo much now and than,*
> *Good diet with wisedome best comforteth man,*
> *In health to be stirring shall profit thee best,*
> *In sickness hate trouble, seeke quiet and reste.*

A Directory for Midwives – Nicholas Culpeper and the Doctrine of Signatures

'No part of medicine is of more general importance than that which relates to the nursing and management of children. Yet few parents pay proper attention to it.' So claimed the famous apothecary Nicholas Culpeper (1616–54) in his *Directory for Midwives* (1651), described as 'a guide for women in their conception, bearing and suckling of their children'. It was the first textbook of its kind to appear in Britain, and it advocated such remedies as a dissolved swallow's nest to speed delivery and the placement of pears in the delivery chamber to delay it.

Culpeper himself was born (presumably without the aid of a

dissolved swallow's nests) in London, just after the death of his father, an ennobled clergyman. At first he attempted to follow in his father's footsteps by reading theology at Cambridge, but he was soon diverted from his studies by his interest in anatomy, medicine and *materia medica*. He failed to graduate and soon moved back to London where he became apprenticed to a master apothecary.

When he was twenty-four he married Alice Field, the daughter of one of his wealthy patients, and she went on to bear him eight children, though only one of them survived into adulthood, a circumstance that perhaps led to his later interest in midwifery. Alice's dowry enabled him to set up his own practice in Spitalfields, and working among the poor Nicholas came to appreciate the necessity of cheap and accessible treatments, in particular those based on herbal medicine. Obtaining his herbs from the surrounding countryside, he was able to treat the poorest patients for free or at little cost. He antagonised both the College of Physicians and the Society of Apothecaries with his radical views about the prevalent medical practice, and at one point he referred to those physicians who charged exorbitant fees for their nostrums as 'bloodsuckers, true vampires'. It was a theme to which he would return.

In 1652 Culpeper published a herbal, originally called *The English Physitian*, a hugely influential book that has been in print ever since. It contains elements of Galen's theory of the four 'humours' (black bile, yellow bile, phlegm and blood) and aspects of astrology. It also refers extensively to the Doctrine of Signatures, the theory that God made an imprint on each plant as a sign of its value and purpose. This theory was extremely influential in Western medicine, though originally it was considered to be spiritual philosophy, thanks to Jakob Böhme (1575–1624), a master shoemaker from Görlitz in Germany. Böhme experienced a profound vision in which the link between God and man was made clear to him. The result was a book, *Signatura Rerum: the Signature of All Things*, which was published in the early 1600s. Shortly afterwards, Paracelsus, whom some consider to be the father of modern chemistry, recognised its potential for medical diagnosis.

The Doctrine of Signatures was based on the premise that the colour of plants and their flowers and fruit, the shape of their leaves and roots, and the place where they grow give some indication of their medicinal qualities. There are hundreds of examples, but here are just a few of them:

Scullcap (Scutellaria baicalensis): the flowers of this herb, reputedly one of the best cures for insomnia, resemble the shape of a human skull.

Eyebright (Euphrasia officinalis): this little blue flower has a yellow centre, which suggests the human eye. Traditionally, it has been used for tired and strained eyes, and the French even call it casse lunettes *(break-glasses).*

Lungwort (Pulmonaria): the patches on the leaves were thought to resemble a diseased lung, so the plants were used for lung conditions.

St John's wort (Hypericum perforatum): the tiny holes in its leaves allow the sun to shine through, and this herb was – and still is – famous for alleviating depression and other symptoms of SAD (Seasonal Affective Disorder).

Yellow plants and herbs: goldenrod (Solidago), for example, and the flowers of dandelion (Taraxacum officinale), pot marigold

(Calendula officinalis) and celandine (Chelidonium) were often used to treat ailments of the liver, including jaundice.

Red plants: these were believed to have an affinity – or signature – with blood and heart conditions.

Irises: the purple petals were commonly used as a poultice for bruising.

Milk thistle (Silybum marianum): the plant thought to help promote milk flow in nursing mothers.

Walnuts (Juglans): the nuts were presumed to be good for the brain.

Aubergines: these were believed to boost the ovaries.

Poplar (Populus spp.), including quaking aspen (P. tremuloides): the trees in the genus were used for the shakes of palsy.

Maidenhair fern (Adiantum capillus-veneris): the fern was used to make a lotion for the treatment for baldness.

A Curious Herbal – Elizabeth Blackwell

Herbal medicine is the oldest form of medical practice. The British Museum has records of a herbal that was once in the library of Ashurbanipal, king of Assyria (668–626 BC). The best-known writers of herbals were the Greek physician Dioscorides, who wrote *De materia medica* in about 65 BC, and, in Britain, John Gerard (1545–1611/12) and Nicholas Culpeper (1616–54). Gerard's and Culpeper's works are still available in modern paperback versions, although nowadays they are read largely because they are quaint, based as they are on the old Galenic system of humours and incorporating astrology and the Doctrine of Signatures.

From the eighteenth to early twentieth century surprisingly few new herbals appeared in Britain, although traditional medicine continued to flourish, particularly in isolated rural communities, where the cost of an apothecary or doctor was beyond the purses of all but the wealthy. What have survived are some of the handwritten manuals of domestic medicine, mostly written by married women from the middle classes or the aristocracy who continued to be a major source of medicinal advice. In fact, many of their remedies differed little from the treatments used by the physicians and apothecaries of the time. There was one notable exception.

Mention the name Elizabeth Blackwell and most medical historians will instantly think of the extraordinary British-born woman (1821–1910) who became the first medical student in the United States. She graduated in 1849 and then started a long campaign to gain recognition first in the United States and then in Britain. It was a further ten years before she was accepted on the lists of the General Medical Council, but she founded the London School of Medicine for Women and was appointed to the chair of gynaecology there in 1874. However, there was an earlier Elizabeth Blackwell and her story is every bit as fascinating.

This Elizabeth was born about 1700 in Aberdeen, and when she was twenty-eight she married Alexander Blackwell, variously described as a physician and apothecary. When challenged about his qualifications – there is no evidence that he had any formal training – Alexander, with Elizabeth, quickly moved to London, where he set up a printing company. He was then fined for trading without undergoing the necessary apprenticeship, his business was closed down and finally, in 1737, he was sent to debtors' prison.

The family fortunes rested with Elizabeth, who now had a child to support. A gifted artist, she was inspired to create an up-to-date herbal for apothecaries, featuring some of the new species from North and South America that were by then being cultivated at Chelsea Physic Garden. This garden on the banks of the Thames, owned by Sir Hans Sloane (1660–1753), was a place of teaching for apothecaries and physicians. Elizabeth moved nearby and, with the support of the curator, began to draw the plants from life. These beautiful, highly detailed illustrations were then engraved on to copper plates, printed and hand coloured.

The result was two volumes, published in parts between 1737 and 1739, with an endorsement from the Royal College of Physicians: *A Curious Herbal containing five hundred cuts of the most useful plants, which are now used in the practice of physick, to which is added a short description of ye plants and their common uses in physic.*

The book was extremely well received and successful, and it is known that, for instance, Sir Joseph Banks, the famous botanist who sailed around the world with Captain Cook kept a copy in his library. The revenue from the book paid Alexander's fine, and he was duly released from gaol, but within a few years he left for Sweden, where he became embroiled in a court conspiracy that led to his execution for treason. According to Elisabeth Brooke in *Women Healers Through History*, Elizabeth Blackwell then trained in obstetrics with the highly respected Dr Smellie and eventually established her own practice.

A Heroine of the Crimean War
— Mary Seacole

Most people have heard of Florence Nightingale, whose powers of persuasion and skills at administration during the Crimean War changed nursing and public health practice. Fewer have heard of Mary Seacole (1805–81), the extraordinary nurse from Jamaica who, having been rejected by Florence Nightingale, set up her own hospital in the Crimea to treat tropical diseases with herbal and folk medicine.

Mary was born in Jamaica of a Creole mother and Scottish father. Her mother was what Mary describes as a 'doctress', and she inspired and educated her young daughter in the traditional medicine of the West Indies. Mary helped her mother to treat the naval officers and their families based nearby.

Mary was restless and longed to travel. As a young woman she visited London, and on her return to Kingston she faced a cholera epidemic and saw at first hand what treatments were successful. This was to prove useful later in her varied career. After travelling widely in the Caribbean – New Providence, Cuba and Haiti – she returned to Kingston and in 1836 married Edwin Horatio Hamilton Seacole, the godson and possibly a relation of Horatio Nelson, but by 1844 she was a widow.

In 1850 Mary's half-brother moved to Cruces in Panama, and she visited him at the time when there was a major outbreak of cholera. She successfully treated her first patient, and her reputation as a healer grew as the disease gained its dreadful hold in the area.

She charged the rich but treated poor people for free. Mary herself became infected, but she self-administered and managed to survive.

She remained in Cruces, where she opened a hotel and continued to treat patients. After a brief return to Kingston, she went back to Panama, where she provided medical support to a mining company. While she was there she heard the first reports of the casualties from the war in the Crimea, which had broken out in 1853. The war was fought between Britain, France, Sardinia and the Ottoman Empire against Russia. Thousands of troops died of a range of infectious diseases, including cholera, without ever reaching the battlefields, while others succumbed during the fighting, from both their wounds and disease.

Mary was soon on her way to offer her services as a nurse. She approached the War Office in London and asked if she could join Florence Nightingale and her team of nurses. Despite her credentials and experience in treating tropical diseases, Mary was thwarted at every turn, most probably because of her colour, and she decided to travel to the Crimea independently, using her own resources. She took a letter of introduction to Florence Nightingale at her hospital in Scutari, but her offer of help was again refused.

She therefore proceeded to set up her own 'British Hotel' near Balaclava to provide 'comfortable quarters for sick and convalescent officers'. In her autobiography, *Wonderful Adventures of Mrs Seacole in Many Lands* (1857), Mary wrote of treating various conditions, including 'that old acquaintance of mine with whom I had had many a bout in past times – cholera'. There were many cases in the Land Transport Corps hospital that was close to hers, and other patients were soon being referred to her. However, it was her courage in working alongside the army doctors in the field hospitals and going out into the battlefield with her 'bag of bandages', treating wounded men under fire, that won her universal acclaim and the nickname Mother Seacole. She was completely bipartisan, treating not only the British but also French and Sardinian soldiers and even 'the Russian enemy'. She was part of the final assault on Sebastopol in 1855 and was the first woman to enter the city when it fell on 9 September.

Mary was among the last to leave the Crimea after the lengthy peace talks. By this time she was virtually destitute and in poor health. She arrived in London in 1856 and within a matter of months, after an abortive business venture, was declared bankrupt. However, her plight was made known in the press, and a fund was set up. Fundraising events were held, including one benefit festival that drew a crowd of 40,000. In 1860 she visited Jamaica for a period but again returned to London. In her latter years she was much feted, with her marble bust exhibited in the Royal Academy's summer exhibition. She also became personal masseuse to the Princess of Wales who suffered with rheumatism. She died in May 1881.

For many years, Mary's achievements were disregarded and her name was almost forgotten. More recently there has been renewed interest in her contribution both in Britain, where in 2004 she was voted into first place in an online poll of 100 Great Black Britons, and in her homeland of Jamaica, where the headquarters of the Jamaican General Training Nurses Association is now named after her. She was also highlighted in Salman Rushdie's *The Satanic Verses* as the 'hidden black history': 'See, here is Mary Seacole. Who did as much in the Crimea as another magic-lamping lady, but, being dark, could scarce be seen for the flame of Florence's candle.'

A Modern Herbal
— Hilda Leyel and Mrs Maud Grieve

'Botany and medicine came down the ages hand in hand until the seventeenth century; then both arts became scientific, their ways parted, and no new herbals were compiled,' says Hilda Leyel in her introduction to *A Modern Herbal* by Mrs Grieve, which was first published in 1931 by Jonathan Cape.

With the exception of Elizabeth Blackwell's illustrated book, she is probably right. Hilda Leyel was trained in orthodox medicine and was a life governor of St Mary's Hospital and the Royal National Orthopaedic Hospital. However, she had a particular interest in herbalism and botany, and realising that much knowledge was being lost or pushed aside in favour of allopathic drugs, she had devoted herself to herbal research from 1916. In 1927 she founded the Herb Society, then called the Society of Herbalists, and also the Culpeper shop. The society had rooms above the shop, and Mrs Leyel also used the address as consulting rooms for her patients.

She wrote: 'Just before I opened Culpeper House, a list of Mrs Grieve's monographs on herbs came to me through the post. I made her acquaintance, and after examining the pamphlets, thought they might be the nucleus of the much-needed modern herbal. I took the monographs and suggestion to Mr Cape, who agreed to publish them if I would collate and edit them and see that American herbs were also included.'

The two ladies formed a long and very rewarding association.

Maud (sometimes Maude) Grieve was the founder and principal of the Whins' Medicinal and Commercial Herb School and Farm in Chalfont St Peter, Buckinghamshire, which offered training courses in every aspect of the growing, harvesting and preparation of medicinal herbs. Her knowledge of medicinal plants was encyclopaedic, and she was a president of the British Guild of Herb Growers as well as a Fellow of the Royal Horticultural Society.

Mrs Grieve's original pamphlets covered only English herbs, many of which she grew herself in her extensive garden. She had accumulated what Hilda Leyel referred to as a 'vast quantity' of material, and Mrs Leyel's task of editing it was formidable. The result was a four-volume publication covering the medicinal, culinary and cosmetic properties of herbs, their cultivation, history and folklore, along with the properties of many trees. English names as well as the Latin names were used, and the tone was very accessible, making the work of interest to lay people as well as to herbalists. A number of the remedies in it have been included in this book.

There is no record of when Mrs Grieve died, but it is known that Mrs Leyel continued to treat patients until her death in 1957.

Rolfing: Helping Gravity to Help Us
— Dr Ida Rolf

Despite a formidable training in orthodox Western medicine, Ida Rolf (1896–1979) relied on her own instincts and beliefs when she came to solving her personal and close family's health issues, and so founded a new form of musculo-skeletal therapy.

Born in New York, Ida was awarded a PhD in biological chemistry from the College of Physicians and Surgeons of Columbia University in 1920. She spent the next twelve years at the Rockefeller Institute carrying out research in organic chemistry, eventually becoming an associate – a very real accomplishment for a young woman at the time. In 1927 she moved to the Swiss Technical University in Zurich to study mathematics and atomic physics, and during this time she also studied homeopathy.

During the 1930s, on her return to the United States, she sought solutions to her own health problems and those of her two sons. She explored osteopathy, chiropractic medicine, yoga and the Alexander technique, and she came to believe that the body functions best when the skeleton is in proper alignment and that any imbalances are reflected in the body's network of soft tissues (muscles, tissues, fascia and tendons). Her life's work developed from the theory of what she called 'structural integration', leading to a system of soft tissue manipulation now known as rolfing. She said: 'This is the gospel of rolfing: when the body gets working appropriately, the force of gravity can flow through. Then, spontaneously, the body heals itself.'

Initially she built a practice in Manhattan, and her reputation quickly spread. In the 1950s and 1960s she started to visit Britain and later California, and soon she was training instructors, making it necessary for her to give a formal structure to her growing organisation. In 1977 she wrote *Rolfing: The Integration of Human Structures*, which laid out her vision, and by the time of her death in 1979 her Guild of Structural Integration had become internationally renowned. Now, there are more than 1,300 Rolf practitioners working in private practice worldwide.

She Stoops to Conker
– The WI and the Home Front

In the hard, grim days of the Second World War maintaining food supplies was an issue of great national concern. As the blockade of Britain by German U-boats tightened, food became increasingly scarce and people were encouraged to grow as much produce as possible in their gardens and allotments. But it wasn't just food that was in short supply. Before the war Britain had imported much of its medical materials – some references suggest up to 90 per cent – in order to manufacture drugs. Germany itself had been a major source of pharmaceutical materials, but once hostilities broke out, this was no longer available. Another supplier, France, was also soon sealed off, as was the Far East. Britain then considered its more distant but friendly suppliers, such as India, South Africa and the Caribbean, but bringing supplies from these distances was not only costly in terms of shipping but also dangerous because of the German blockade. The government realised that the country would quickly face a serious shortage of vital drugs unless local alternatives could be found.

During the First World War the Ministry of Agriculture and Fisheries had asked people to collect herbs for drug manufacture. While the response had been immediate and enthusiastic, it had had limited effect because frequently the herbs were incorrectly dried and stored or had been mixed up, making them of no value.

Aware of this, in June 1941 the Minister of Health created a specialist committee to consider how herbs could best be harvested from across Britain. The initiative soon became the responsibility of the Vegetable Drugs Committee, part of the Ministry of Supply, which looked at two distinct groups: a long-term group that would grow plants from new seed, which would, therefore, take several years to establish, and a short-term group that would be responsible for increasing current production and gathering wild plants.

The response was the formation of herb committees in every county in the country, thirty-eight in all. It was also agreed that collecting herbs would be classed as 'work of national importance', and drug manufacturers were asked to supply lists of the plants they required. Posters, media publicity and short films were produced to promote the mission.

Members of the Women's Institute (WI) were recruited as principal collectors, backed by Boy Scouts and Girl Guides. Local schoolchildren were drafted in, and in some areas the women of the Land Army were also recruited. By the 1940s about 80,000 women volunteers worked on the land for minimal wages, replacing the men who had gone to fight. Juliette de Bairacli Levy, who was to become an internationally renowned herbalist, author and traveller, famous for pioneering holistic veterinary medicine, recalls gathering sphagnum moss – used to make dressings – during her time in the Land Army. (The use and properties of sphagnum moss are described under Cuts and wounds.)

The Scouts were asked to collect nettles, dandelion roots, colchicum (meadow saffron) and foxgloves. WI members were given a crash course by way of lectures with lantern slides on the identification, drying and storage of herbs. They were given a slightly wider remit than the Scouts, and their list included belladonna leaves, colchicum leaves and seeds, foxglove leaves and seeds (to make digitalin, used in the treatment of heart disease), male fern rhizome (used to treat worms), valerian root (an anti-spasmodic), coltsfoot (for bronchial complaints), broom tops (for treating high blood pressure) and certain seaweeds used to produce agar jelly from which penicillin could be derived.

They were also required to collect horse chestnuts, which could be made into Leucozade, widely prescribed by doctors as a glucose drink. This gave rise to a number of cartoons in the WI publications under such headings as 'She Stoops to Conker'.

Most famously, the WI spearheaded the campaign to collect rosehips, which were discovered to have three to four times as much vitamin C as blackcurrants and twenty times that of oranges, now anyway in short supply. Once made into a syrup, rosehips made a very acceptable alternative for children. A target of 2,000 tons was set for 1943, and whole communities were recruited to help with collection, including evacuees. Norman Drysdale, who was evacuated from Glasgow to Bentham in Lancashire, remembers that one of his tasks was to gather rosehips from the hedgerows and that these would be collected in sacks and taken 'to make vitamin C for city children'. Marguerite Hughes, whose family moved to Malvern in Worcestershire to escape the bombing in London, also recalls collecting rosehips. She joined the local WI when she was fourteen years old and cannot remember whether it was a WI initiative or through her local school. Meanwhile, Margaret Paxton, who as a child lived at Blindcrake, near Cockermouth in Cumbria, would collect rosehips on her way to and from school in Isel. She was given 3d – three old pennies – per pound.

In January 1942 in the 'News of the Month' section of *Home & Country*, the WI magazine, there was a report headed 'Medicinal Herbs':

> *One firm alone paid out £1,500 for herbs collected by WI members last year and would willingly have paid for fifteen times the amount collected. Improved coordination this year should see that that urgent demand should be satisfied. So long as proper care is taken in picking, so that the source of supply is maintained, valuable drugs can be provided and some useful weeding done in one stroke!*

In August 1942 the Isle of Wight WI gave notice of a public meeting it was hoping to hold, inviting all organisations, including the Girl Guides and Boy Scouts, to discuss how herbs could be collected locally. By October of the same year the minutes noted: 'Rosehips are urgently wanted, also horse chestnuts, for medicinal purposes.' But it was the WI Federation of Leicester and Rutland that finally won a national award for collecting the greatest weight of rosehips.

By 1943 Britain was importing only 50 per cent of the quantity of medicinal herbs and plants that it had imported before the outbreak of war, a considerable achievement considering that the scheme was only in its third year.

A Traveller's Tale – Annie Penfold

It is amazing how many remedies are reportedly given to women 'by a gypsy', and the phenomenon is recounted several times in this book. There is clearly an underlying belief that travellers had access to cures and treatments that the more static communities did not. Maybe there is the hope that a gypsy had special powers of foresight – or was in some way closer to intuitive elements.

Annie Penfold believes in fresh air, fresh food, hard work – and salt! At the time of writing, Annie is ninety-three years old, has seven children, eighteen grandchildren, thirty-nine great-grandchildren and, currently, two great-great-grandchildren. With the exception of a short time when she was first married, Annie has lived all her life in a caravan, and it is partly to this that she attributes her longevity and continued energy. Both her parents were gypsies, and her early life was spent travelling all over England. Her parents too lived long and healthy lives, her father living until he was ninety-seven.

'We've always lived out in the fresh air, with fresh food often plucked straight from the ground, and we've worked hard physically too. This is the way to stay healthy,' she explains. She lived in a house for a while but didn't enjoy it. Even then she spent five months of the year working in the fields, picking flowers, fruit, vegetables and hops. Life was hard, but she is unsentimental about its toughness.

Her husband, Arthur, ran a florist stall on the Fulham Road in London for many years, and Annie will tell you about the celebrities among his customers: Margot Fonteyn, Charlie Chaplin ('He wrote to cancel his flower order when he moved to America but I've lost the letter over the years'), the artist Jacob Epstein, the murderer John Christie and on to a younger set, including Sir Paul McCartney and Cilla Black. Arthur's mother, Lily, achieved her own fame: she was painted by the great Chelsea artist, Augustus John.

Annie brought up her family on simple tried and tested remedies. She would bring a child's temperature down by bathing them in cold water. Cuts were stitched with cotton or held together with plaster. Salt was used as an antiseptic, and hot water was considered the best remedy for digestive problems. She still has a beautiful complexion, which she attributes to washing in cold water – and she continues to take the occasional cold water bath. Visiting a doctor or going to hospital were the last resorts, certainly not the first, and her family still subscribes to this philosophy. Her granddaughter believes that people nowadays are afraid to put up with a bit of discomfort.

Nowadays, the family lives on an established, well-ordered site in Merton, southwest London. Annie's family surround her, but despite that she continues to do her own gardening and shopping. 'Always fresh meat, dear, we don't have processed foods or keep meat in a deep freezer. And always drink the water you have boiled the vegetables in, or at least use it to make gravy,' she insists. Here are some of Annie's remedies:

For cuts, open the wound and wash with salt water. For smaller cuts, hold the edges together with plasters, then there's no need for stitching.

Dandelions are good for sore throats and coughs. Boil them, strain them and drink the juice.

Cut a potato in half and rub it on a burn. The best things come out of the ground.

Use a compress of tealeaves to bring down the swelling of an ankle.

Use honey or salt in water as a gargle for a sore throat.

Chew a stick of chalk – the kind used for writing on a blackboard – for heartburn.

West to East – *Anne McIntyre*

Anne McIntyre has had a lifelong passion for plants. Even as a small child she grew flowers – pansies, daffodils and antirrhinums – in her own tiny patch of garden. Her fascination continues undiminished, and she believes herself to be on a ladder of learning.

Her 'patch' now is a herb garden in the beautiful village of Great Rissington, Gloucestershire, where hundreds of plants grow in ordered abundance. The garden – which is open to the public for guided tours – has been created to the form of a woman's journey, starting with a tunnel that represents the birth canal, surrounded by the herbs that facilitate birth and settle a new baby. A spiral path takes visitors on the lifetime of healing and maintenance, through childhood diseases to the onset of menses. There are grottos representing the times of love, marriage and fertility, followed by a path representing the period of high activity, as women make homes, bring up their children and build their careers. The spiral leads round to menopause and the time when women become wiser and pay attention to more spiritual matters. Finally, the spiral concludes in an exquisite round pond, with a fountain that springs from a sculpted lotus flower. This and the herbs that surround it represent eternal life.

Anne became intrigued by Buddhism when she was sixteen. She had been given a book called *The Wisdom of India*, which contained many ancient texts, and she took a local Buddhist meditation class and befriended her teacher. She elected to take Eastern religion and Sanskrit at university and spent a year in India as soon as her exams were over.

On her return to Britain, she had a strong urge to find out how people in this country could live in harmony with the natural world. She moved to a cottage by herself on a small island off the Essex coast, where she became self-sufficient, exploring and collecting wild things to see how they could heal the body, mind and spirit. She decided to take her studies of herbal medicine further, persuading her local authority to give her a grant to undertake a course at the School of Herbal Medicine in Tunbridge Wells.

Eventually, at the age of twenty-seven, Anne began to see patients. She added further training, at first in massage, and then in aromatherapy, which she saw as a bridge between massage and herbalism. She took a course in counselling so she could understand better and at a deeper level the imbalances that are created between the mind and the body. Still not satisfied, she also trained in homeopathy, so she would understand dosage and the potency of herbal tinctures. She explains her approach:

> Every herb has a healing force. In some ways, it doesn't matter how you use it, whether as an oil, an essence, a tincture or in a homeopathic dosage. Sometimes you just need to be in its presence. For example, if you were to look at a beautiful rose right at this moment, you would probably smile. Just the sight of it – and its aroma – would be beneficial. I am fascinated not just by the biochemistry of a plant but also its energies.
>
> I am wary of herbalists who only give standard formulas and would warn patients against them. I make tailor-made formulas, designed for each specific patient, their constitution, mindset and approach to life.

It was at this time that she learned that Dr Vasant Ladd, the world-renowned expert on Ayurvedic medicine, was conducting a short course in Britain, and she rushed to sign up. In this she found what she had been searching for: 'the bridge between my love of Eastern philosophy and my practice as a medical herbalist. I have huge confidence in Ayurveda as a framework. After all it has 5,000 years of ancient wisdom to support it!'

Even now Anne firmly believes that on many levels she is still studying, but, she says: 'I used to give remedies with hope. Now I give them with a sense of knowing. I have been a herbalist for twenty-six years and I now teach at the Scottish School of Herbal Medicine and in the United States. But it isn't just learned experience, I draw on all the disciplines and an understanding of how patients' minds and bodies interrelate.'

Anne has written a number of beautiful and authoritative books, which have found ready audiences in many countries. In addition to her masterwork, *The Complete Floral Healer*, she has written a herbal for women, and a book of herbal treatments for children. Nowadays, she divides her time between Gloucestershire with her garden, her clinic and her family and London and her teaching commitments.

Following in Grandma's Footsteps

If you would like to help preserve the long tradition of women as guardians of family health by becoming part of it, the following pages offer some practical advice. You could devote your own kitchen garden – no matter how small – to growing medicinal and culinary herbs, or create a store of preparations in the form of teas, tinctures, syrups, tonics, glycerites and ointments to treat minor everyday ailments.

Starting a herb garden

Nowadays, with so many different herbs available in garden centres, both in containers and as seeds, home cultivation is simple. It doesn't even require a garden or a balcony. A hanging basket can hold a number of different herbs, as can windowboxes and other containers, such as troughs, stone jars, terracotta pots and even old watering cans. If none of these opportunities is available to you, consider joining a community or city farm project or putting your name down for an allotment.

Whether you are growing plants in a patch in the garden or in a few containers, aim to keep them in a sheltered but sunny position. Make sure that the ground is well drained, and if you are using containers put a good layer of stones or gravel in the bottom before you add an organic soil mixture. In general, the more space there is around each plant, the bigger it is likely to grow, but be careful of plants like mint (*Mentha*) and lovage (*Levisticum*), which spread all too easily. Restrict their roots by growing them in an old bucket or bowl with the bottom knocked out that you can sink into the ground.

Herbs are annual, biennial or perennial. If you are growing herbs in containers, you might prefer to keep annuals together in one pot, biennials in other and so on, simply because it is easier to re-pot them later on.

Plant in spring, trim during summer and cut back herbaceous perennials (those that die back to the ground) in autumn. Evergreen herbs, such as rosemary, should be pruned lightly in spring. If you can, move containers to a sheltered place over winter, and in severe weather consider sheltering them in a garage or shed because the roots of plants in containers are much more at risk of freezing than those of plants growing in the ground.

In spring and summer water and feed your herbs regularly. Be aware of pests such as slugs and snails. One solution is to grow yarrow (*Achillea*) and camomile (*Chamaemelum*) nearby, which slugs do not like. But both slugs and snails have an extraordinary ability to defeat many would-be deterrents, although by all means try edging plants with borders of hair or crushed glass or whatever is the latest wheeze.

Selecting your herbs

The temperate climate of Britain has always been exceptionally good for growing a huge range of herbs and beneficial plants. We can derive some idea of the herbs that were grown in monastic or convent herb gardens in the Middle Ages from the one at Gloucester Cathedral. This was re-established in the 1990s close to where the infirmary had been sited between about 1150 and 1540. It has been reinstated with loving care, and you can visit it today.

The herb garden contains four main types of herbs: medicinal; strewing and cosmetic; dyeing and fumigating; and culinary. Medicinal herbs included lovage, feverfew, marjoram, marsh mallow, St John's wort, rue, box and fennel.

Among the strewing and cosmetic herbs were rosemary, lavender, sweet cicely, vervain, violet and primroses, meadowsweet, soapwort, fennel and curry plant. Herbs for dyeing and fumigating included dyer's madder and dyer's greenweed, woad, pot marigold, teasels, hyssop, hemp agrimony, and wormwood and southern wood. The culinary herbs were parsley, fennel, sweet cicely, bay, thyme, bergamot, sage and mint.

Most of these species are still in use and are widely available today, although you may not need those for dyeing nor, hopefully, those for fumigating. Many are also sold as improved forms, which are even better suited to temperate climates and which have coloured flowers or variegated foliage.

If you have limited space, you might opt for the more popular herbs: rosemary, lavender, fennel, sage, parsley, marjoram, camomile, basil and thyme. Add some nasturtiums or sunflowers for colour, and remember that you can use these in cooking and for teas and tinctures. If you have more space in your garden you could consider planting a wider range of herbs and beneficial plants. Try garlic, onions, roses – both for the flowers and for rosehips – raspberries, pot marigolds, valerian, feverfew and watercress (if you have a clear stream), and don't forget to leave some of the 'weeds' such as dandelions, nettles and evening primroses. The list is long. However, there has been a greater interest in herb growing in recent years, and many of the larger garden centres employ specialists in this area, who can give you advice on what will grow best in the type of soil in your garden, and what will grow in shade or in direct sunlight.

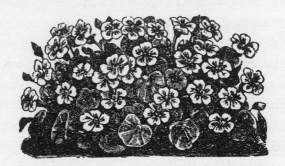

Nasturtiums will add colour to any herb garden, and are a great source of vitamin C

Harvesting

A herb grown in one kind of soil and climate will differ in the strength of its properties from the same species grown under different conditions. In addition, herbs may well vary in quality and quantity from season to season.

While there are a lot of strange myths surrounding the times and procedures for gathering herbs – the need to go barefoot or to gather them by the light of the moon and so on – it does make sense to harvest them when the plant is at a suitable horticultural stage, so that the essential constituents are at their highest concentration.

Usually the best time to collect a herb for drying is when the plant is at its peak, in full growth but just before it blooms. This is the stage when the plant's nutrients and oils are mainly concentrated in its leaves. There is no need to uproot the plants unless you are harvesting bulbs, such as onions, or roots, such as horseradish (*Armoracia rusticana*). Instead, you should harvest them by snipping off shoots with a sharp knife or a pair of scissors to prevent bruising. Collect sprigs rather than individual leaves, so that you do not handle the delicate leaves and stems you are drying and also do no harm to the parent plant.

It is best to collect herbs in dry weather – wet herbs may develop mildew during drying – and you should aim to gather them before the sun is up or, at the very least, before the dew has evaporated. This will ensure that maximum moisture, aroma and goodness are held in the petals and leaves before the sun dries them and leeches them away.

To maintain their colour and flavour, prepare the herbs for drying as soon as possible. Lay them down carefully: a shallow basket is ideal. Piling them on top of one another may again cause bruising. Fruits and seeds can be collected but only when they are fully ripe. Roots and bulbs should be gathered in autumn and winter.

If you are gathering wild herbs, do not collect them from near busy roadsides, where they have been exposed to exhaust fumes and may have absorbed lead, or close to fields, where pesticides and chemical fertilisers may have been used.

Drying and storing

Ideally, herbs should be dried as quickly as possible. This means keeping them in a moderately warm place with a good circulation of air. Do not try to dry them in direct sunlight, because this will bleach the colour. Dry, well-ventilated garden sheds are ideal, or you could use understairs cupboards or even airing cupboards as long as the doors can be left slightly ajar to allow air to circulate freely. Herbs will absorb any strong smells around them, so busy kitchens and garages are less ideal, and any dampness in the atmosphere is likely to cause the growth of mould. Jamie Oliver suggests that a ledge or shelf above the oven can be a good place, but be prepared for your herbs to take on the fragrances of your cooking. Be aware, too, that steam from your saucepans can make them mouldy.

Hang up larger herbs in bunches, attaching the bunches to wire coathangers or looping them on butcher's hooks. Spread out smaller herbs on wire racks. If you want, line the rack with paper, linen, a tea towel or muslin. You might like to cover the herbs lightly too, to keep flies and insects away.

If you are drying leaves, wipe off any soil or debris but try to avoid washing them. Herbs with small leaves should be dried flat. Turn them gently each day so that all parts of the plant are exposed to the air and warmth. Once the leaves are dry and slightly brittle, and the stems break rather than bend, they are ready for use.

Flowers can be dried in the same way. Handle them carefully to avoid damaging and marring the petals. Properly dried, they should be slightly crisp. Leave seed- and flowerheads, such as lavender, attached to the stems, enclose them in paper bags (not plastic) and hang them upside down. They will dry quite quickly.

All roots should be scrubbed and fibrous parts cut away before drying. You can split large, tough roots down the centre or cut them into small pieces to speed the drying process. Again, you will need to turn them regularly. Bark may need gentle washing to remove moss and insects before being dried in a dark, warm place.

Drying normally takes two to three weeks. If you want to keep the herbs for some time, transfer them to small, airtight containers. Dark glass bottles and jars are best. Avoid plastic containers, which may encourage sweating. Don't forget to add labels, showing not only the name of the plant but also the date on which it was harvested. Store in a dark, dry place.

Some people suggest using a microwave oven to dry herbs, but not all herbalists subscribe to this method. If you try it, be careful that you don't overcook the herbs. Check that the herb of your choice has retained its flavour if you use this method because not all will do so.

Some herbs can be frozen, including chives, parsley, tarragon, sorrel and mint. However, camomile, thyme, rosemary, marigold, feverfew and savory are not suitable. Some people like to blanch herbs before freezing, but others find this process unnecessary. Drop the herb in a plastic bag and put it in the freezer, where it should keep its qualities for up to six months. You can also chop the herbs and drop them into a little water in the sections of ice-cube trays, which makes it easier to add just a small quantity at any one time.

Another way to preserve herbs that is particularly appropriate if you are going to use them for massage or in cookery is to put them in oils or vinegars. Make sure that the leaves and stems are perfectly dry, put them in a clean glass bottle or jar, add good quality vegetable oil or vinegar and seal tightly. Keep in a cool dark place.

Preparing herbs for use

The herbs you have collected, whether freshly harvested or dried, can be prepared in many ways for medicinal use. The flavour of fresh herbs is always preferable, and it is good to see that such a wide range is now sold in markets and supermarkets. Bear in mind when you use dried herbs that their flavour has been concentrated during the drying process, and they will be two to three times the strength of the flavour of the fresh equivalent.

Dried herbs and spices are also best used as quickly as possible after harvesting. Keep them in airtight jars in a dry, dark cupboard or larder, away from sunlight, and use them within about six months.

Making an INFUSION

You make an infusion from either fresh or dried herbs taken from the soft parts of the plant – that is, the flowers, thin stems or leaves. Chop or snip them into pieces or use the sprigs whole. If you are using whole sprigs crush them slightly with a spoon to release their goodness and flavour. If they are dried it doesn't matter whether they are loose or in a teabag. Warm a teapot by rinsing it in hot water, and put in one dessertspoonful of dried herb for every cup required. Double the quantity if you are using fresh herbs.

Herbalists will suggest that you boil water and then allow it to go off the boil before pouring over your herbs. Use freshly drawn water or even bottled mineral water if you live in an area where the tapwater is very hard. Allow the mixture to steep for 10–15 minutes, then strain (if necessary) and drink the infusion as soon as it is cool enough or cover and store it in a cool place for up to 48 hours. It is usual to drink herbal teas without milk or sugar, but you can use a little honey as a sweetener if the herb is bitter.

A tisane (tea) is a mild version of an infusion. Add fresh or dried herbs to boiling water and drink as soon as it is cool enough, without steeping.

Making a DECOCTION

A decoction is appropriate when you want to release the properties from the tougher parts of a plant – that is, from the bark, seeds or roots.

Place 10 oz (300 g) of powdered dried herbs or 1 lb 3 oz (600 g) of fresh herbs in cold water in a stainless steel or enamel saucepan.

Do not use an aluminium container. Make sure that the plant parts of fresh herbs are crushed or bruised so that their properties are more easily extracted. Bring the water to the boil and simmer for at least 15 minutes or until the liquid has reduced by about a quarter. Strain through muslin and either drink right away or store in a cool place for up to 48 hours.

You will notice the distinctive difference between a decoction and an infusion and one that early herbalists, including North American Indians identified. An infusion is prepared by extracting the beneficial qualities of the material after the water has boiled. A decoction requires actively boiling water to extract the qualities.

Making a TINCTURE

A tincture is a concentrated extract of a specific herb. Making tinctures allows you to store medicinal herbs for long periods by preserving them in a mixture of water and alcohol, avoiding the necessity to make a fresh batch every day or so. If possible, make the tincture from fresh herbs and chop them as you would if you were making a tea.

Place 8 oz (250 g) of fresh herbs or 4 oz (125 g) of dried herbs in a container – a glass jar is perfect – with a tight-fitting top. Add 1 pint (600 ml) of liquid, part pure water, part alcohol (such as brandy, gin or vodka). Make sure that the alcohol is at least 40 per cent proof. The ratio of water to alcohol can differ according to the remedy you are preparing. Anne McIntyre suggests that 25 per cent alcohol would be sufficient for a glycerite (see page 226), while 90 per cent alcohol is necessary for resins and gums.

Seal the jar and keep it in a warm dark place for two weeks, shaking it twice a day. Strain through muslin or use a wine press to squeeze out the liquid before discarding the herb. Decant the tincture into a dark glass bottle, and remember to add a label with both the name of the herb and the date you made it. A properly made tincture will keep for up to two years if kept away from heat and light.

Tinctures are highly concentrated, so they should be taken in small doses. The usual dosage for adults is a teaspoon (5 ml) three times a day, taken with or without food for chronic conditions and taken every two hours for acute conditions. Halve the dosage for children and old people.

Making a SYRUP

Most people in Britain over the age of forty-five will have taken a medicinal syrup at some time. People born just after the Second World War, the so-called baby boomers, will be acquainted with rosehip syrup, which provided them with vitamin C (see page 97), and they may even have been given syrup of figs for constipation. In fact, a syrup can be made from any infusion, decoction or tincture in order to make it more palatable, particularly for children.

A syrup is quite simply a concentrated solution of sugar (or honey) to which the medicinal constituent of the herb is added. There are three basic methods:

Using 12 oz (375 g) of sugar to 1 pint (600 ml) of the decoction or infusion. Heat until the sugar dissolves and the consistency becomes syrupy.

Alternatively, take equal parts of heated honey and the medicinal decoction or infusion, and mix them.

Finally, boil 1 pint (600 ml) of water, pour it over 2½ lb (1.25 kg) of sugar and return to a low heat until the sugar has dissolved. Remove from the heat once it has boiled and allow the syrup to cool, then add one part of tincture to three parts of the syrup.

Making a GLYCERITE

A glycerite (or glycerol) is an alternative to a tincture, made by extracting herbs using glycerine. This is particularly useful for people who cannot tolerate or do not want to take herbal preparations containing alcohol. Glycerites mix well with other liquids, such as fruit juice or sweet oils. Most glycerines are made from animal fats, but if you are a vegetarian you can find one made from a vegetable source, such as coconut oil.

The basic ingredients are 3½ oz (100 g) of finely chopped herbs, 1 pint (600 ml) of glycerine (minimum 60 per cent by volume) and 11 fl oz (325 ml) of distilled water. Put the herbs in a glass jar. Mix together the glycerine and distilled water and pour over the herbs. Leave to macerate for two weeks, shaking the jar daily.

Making an OINTMENT

It is relatively simple, if time consuming, to make ointments or salves at home. In the past the chosen fat was often lard, but in these cholesterol-conscious days, people usually prefer to use a pure vegetable oil, such as olive or sunflower.

You will need 4 oz (125 g) of fresh herbs or 2 oz (50 g) of dried herbs, 1 pint (600 ml) of olive or sunflower oil and 1–1½ oz (25–40 g) of beeswax. Heat the oil and herbs gently for 1–1½ hours in an uncovered container, so that the plant's healing properties are fully absorbed. You can use a bain-marie (a heatproof bowl standing in a larger saucepan of water). Add the beeswax to the mixture as it heats. Strain the mixture by pressing through muslin and pour the warm oil into glass jars to solidify.

If you want a runnier ointment simply increase the amount of beeswax in the recipe. Another, more modern method is to stir a tincture, infusion or decoction into a scoop of aqueous cream, which you can find in most pharmacies.

Making a LINIMENT

Liniments are applied to the skin, and they contain herb extracts that have been added either to oil or to rubbing alcohol. In the past liniments were more quaintly referred to as embrocations and were used on animals, particularly horses, as well as humans. They were – and sometimes still are – used for massage to relieve the pain of aching joints, sprains, sore muscles and other injuries. The skin quickly absorbs the liniment, and sometimes it will react slightly, turning red. Before using a liniment for the first time, therefore, you should apply a small amount, perhaps to your wrist, to test it.

A typical liniment can be made from 3½ oz (100 g) of herbs (these may be a mixture) and 2 pints (1.2 litres) of rubbing alcohol. Mix together the herbs and alcohol and allow to stand for seven days, shaking the mixture well once a day. Decant and pour into glass bottles and add a stopper or cork. Tinctures made from alcohol can also be added to a liniment.

Remember that liniments are for external use only and should never be swallowed.

Making a POULTICE

Poultices are made by placing a beneficial substance directly on the skin or between pieces gauze. They are usually warmed or else they are by their nature warming. Poultices are sometimes used to ease pain or bring out infections, such as sores, carbuncles or boils. They were also used in cases of acute disease to keep vital organs or muscle groups from becoming chilled. Traditionally, poultices were made mostly of bread, sometimes mashed in hot milk, hot water or even boiled with vinegar to make a paste. Oatmeal was also used, again made into a paste by mixing it with water. Excess moisture was squeezed out of the paste so it became a more malleable pad. Another type of poultice that was available from pharmacies was made from kaolin, which would then be heated before being applied.

Nowadays, we use poultices mainly to treat boils and localised infections. It is most likely that soothing herbs, such as slippery elm (*Ulmus rubra*) or comfrey root (*Symphytum* spp.), are used to draw out pus and reduce inflammation.

The usual method is to make the dried herbs of your choice into a paste with very hot water, and to place it directly on the site of the infection, holding it in position with a gauze bandage. Take care, because some dried herbs placed directly on the skin can cause irritation. If you have sensitive skin lay the paste on a piece of gauze first. Maintain the heat by holding a hot water bottle to the poultice.

Freshly cut herbs can also be used, and these can be placed directly on the skin or held in position between pieces of gauze.

Other good poultices can be made from honey, which has antiseptic qualities (just spread it over an infected area) or bacon fat. You can also use onions. Bake the onion first and place it over the boil or infected area. Alternatively, chop up the onion, cover it with salt, leave it overnight and then strain. Use the onion juice, which has antiseptic properties.

Making a COMPRESS

Compresses can be used either hot or cold, depending on the condition to be treated. Take a clean piece of linen or cotton, towelling or even cotton wool. Soak it in a very hot infusion or decoction, then wring it out. Place the cloth on the area to be treated and bind it in position with a bandage, a length of cloth or even cling film. For a hot compress place a towel over the area to keep in the heat or hold a hot water bottle over the compress.

A cold compress is useful when there is swelling – a twisted ankle, for example – or to cool fever or a 'hot' headache. It is made in just the same way, by soaking fabric in an appropriate infusion and allowing it to cool before applying.

Jack of the nursery rhyme was quite possibly treated with a compress:

> *Jack and Jill went up the hill*
> *To fetch a pail of water,*
> *Jack fell down and broke his crown,*
> *And Jill came tumbling after.*
>
> *Up Jack got and home he ran,*
> *As fast as he could caper.*
> *There his mother bound his head,*
> *With vinegar and brown paper.*

Making a FOMENTATION

Compresses can be either hot or cold depending on the condition being treated, but hot and cold fomentations are used alternately in one treatment.

Use either infusions or decoctions as you would for a compress (see above). The hot fomentation should be applied as hot as the patient can stand, although you should test it first to make sure it is not scalding. Once applied, the fomentation should be covered in towels to retain the heat. A fomentation is normally applied for between fifteen minutes and an hour. The aim of the fomentation is to stimulate circulation or to aid congestion in the body or to bring down swellings. See, for example, Back pain on page 12.

Places to Visit

Acorn Bank Garden and Watermill

Temple Sowerby
near Penrith
Cumbria CA10 1SP
Tel: 01768 361 893
www.nationaltrust.org.uk
An incredibly well-stocked herb garden with more than 250 medicinal and culinary varieties.

Bristol Chinese Herb Garden

University of Bristol Botanic
Garden
The Holmes
Stoke Park Road
Stoke Bishop
Bristol BS8 1JB
Tel: 0117 331 4912
www.rchm.co.uk/BCHG.htm
This garden is the result of a partnership between the University of Bristol Botanic Garden and the Register of Chinese Herbal Medicine. Founded in 2000 and expanded in 2006, it aims to provide a comprehensive living collection of the plants used in traditional Chinese medicine.

Calke Abbey

Ticknall
Derbyshire DE73 7LE
Tel: 01332 863 822
www.nationaltrust.org.uk
Dating from the eighteenth century, Calke's garden was created for the cultivation of medicinal herbs and plants.

Chartwell

Mapleton Road
Westerham
Kent TN16 1PS
Tel: 01732 866368
www.nationaltrust.org.uk
*Winston Churchill's family home
includes a restored vegetable garden
where herbs are also grown.*

Chelsea Physic Garden

66 Royal Hospital Road
London SW3 4HS
Tel: 020 7352 5646
www.chelseaphysicgarden.co.uk
*Established in 1673 by the Society of
Apothecaries, this historic garden has
aided the study of plants' therapeutic
properties for many years.*

Coton Manor Garden

Coton
Northamptonshire NN6 8RQ
Tel: 01604 740219
www.cotonmanor.co.uk
*A peaceful garden in the grounds of
a beautiful seventeenth-century manor
house.*

Droitwich Spa Lido

St Andrews Road
Droitwich Spa
Worcestershire WR9 8DN
Tel: 01905 793446
www.brinebath.co.uk
*The brine at this spa is pumped from
an underground lake 200 feet below
the town and is the strongest natural
saltwater known, ten times more
concentrated than normal seawater.
The original baths were built by the
Victorians and can still be enjoyed
today.*

Felbrigg Hall, Garden and Park

Felbrigg
Norwich
Norfolk NR11 8PR
Tel: 01263 837 444
www.nationaltrust.org.uk
*This impressive Stuart house has
a charming walled kitchen garden.*

Garden Organic

Ryton
Coventry
Warwickshire CV8 3LG
Tel: 024 7630 3517
www.gardenorganic.org.uk
Here you can see organic display gardens belonging to the leading charity for organic growing.

Glasgow Cathedral

Castle Street
Glasgow G4 0QZ
Tel: 0141 552 8198
www.glasgowcathedral.org.uk
In the cathedral precinct, restored in the mid-1990s, is a re-creation of the ancient St Nicholas Physic Garden, a medieval herb garden.

Gloucester Cathedral

2 College Green
Gloucester GL1 2LR
Tel: 01452 528095
www.gloucestercathedral.org.uk
Like many medieval cathedrals that were attached to monasteries, Gloucester has a herb garden that can be visited. It was re-established in the 1990s close to where the infirmary, which existed between about 1150

and 1540, had been sited. The herb garden has four main types of herbs: medicinal; strewing and cosmetic; dyeing and fumigating; and culinary.

Kelmscott Manor

Kelmscott
Lechlade
Gloucestershire GL7 3HJ
Tel: 01367 252486
www.kelmscottmanor.co.uk
This grade 1 listed Tudor farmhouse was the country home of the craftsman-poet William Morris and has a thriving herb garden.

Loseley Park

Estate Office
Guildford
Surrey GU3 1HS
Tel: 01483 304440
www.loseley-park.com
Loseley Park's herb garden contains a fascinating array of over 200 herbs categorised in four separate areas: culinary, medicinal, household and decorative.

National Botanic Garden of Wales

Llanarthne
Carmarthenshire SA32 8HG
Tel: 01558 668768
www.gardenofwales.org.uk
This relatively new garden was created in 2000 and features an exhibition dedicated to the physicians of Myddfai as well as an Apothecaries' Hall and an Apothecaries' Garden.

Norton Priory Museum and Gardens

Tudor Road
Manor Park
Runcorn
Cheshire WA7 1SX
Tel: 01928 569895
www.nortonpriory.org
The 2½ acre walled garden was built between 1757 and 1770 for the Brooke family, then owners of Norton Priory. It has now been re-created as a typical Georgian kitchen garden.

Norwich Cathedral

12 The Close
Norwich NR1 4DH
Tel: 01603 218300
www.cathedral.org.uk

Benedictine monks had extensive knowledge of plants and their uses. A new herb garden was created in 2002 close to the site of the original monastic garden.

Roman Baths

Abbey Church Yard
Bath BA1 1LZ
Tel: 01225 477785
www.romanbaths.co.uk
A fascinating building where you can see how the baths were used from Roman times through to the present day.

Royal Botanic Gardens

Kew
Richmond
Surrey TW9 3AB
Tel: 020 8332 5655
www.kew.org
Thanks to a succession of avid collectors, visionary scientists and inspired landscape architects, the Royal Botanic Gardens at Kew are a World Heritage Site and a joy to visit.

Royal College of Physicians

11 St Andrews Place
Regent's Park
London NW1 4LE
Tel: 020 7935 1174
www.rcplondon.ac.uk
*The College's Heritage Centre will
organise tours of the collections by
appointment.*

Royal Pharmaceutical
Society Museum

1 Lambeth High Street
London SE1 7JN
Tel: 020 7572 2210
www.rpsgb.org.uk/
informationresources/museum/
*This museum collection was started
in 1842 and now contains over 45,000
items covering all aspects of British
pharmaceutical history.*

Royal Pump Rooms

The Parade
Royal Leamington Spa
Warwickshire CV32 4AA
Tel: 01926 742700
www.royal-pump-rooms.co.uk
*An art gallery and museum in a
converted swimming pool and Turkish
bath.*

Sissinghurst Castle Garden

Sissinghurst
near Cranbrook
Kent TN17 2AB
Tel: 01580 710701
www.nationaltrust.org.uk
*One of the world's most celebrated
gardens, created by Vita Sackville-
West and her husband Sir Harold
Nicolson.*

Sulgrave Manor

Manor Road
Sulgrave
near Banbury
Oxfordshire OX17 2SD
Tel: 01295 760205
www.sulgravemanor.org.uk
*Now the headquarters of the Herb
Society, the house dates from 1539
and was the ancestral home of George
Washington's forebears. A herb
garden has been created by the society,
and it contains some of the plants that
the early settlers took to North America
and some of those species that were
brought back.*

Winchester Cathedral

1 The Close
Winchester
Hampshire SO23 9LS
Tel: 01962 857200
www.winchester-cathedral.org.uk
*In the enchanting Dean Garnier
Garden in Cathedral Close, there is a
monks' herb garden, which is planted
with the medicinal herbs that the
Benedictine monks would have used.*

Worshipful Society of Apothecaries

Apothecaries' Hall
Black Friars Lane
London EC4V 6EJ
Tel: 020 7236 1189
www.apothecaries.org
*Visits to the hall are by appointment
only.*

Bibliography & Further Reading

Allardice, Pamela, *A–Z of Essential Oils*, Lansdowne Press, Sydney, 1994

Brooke, Elisabeth, *Women Healers Through History*, The Women's Press, London, 1993

Costley, Sarah, and Knightly, Charles, *A Celtic Book of Days*, Thames & Hudson, London, 1998

Culpeper, Nicholas, *Complete Herbal*, 1653 (reprinted Wordsworth Reference, 1995)

Elliot, Rose, and De Paoli, Carlo, *The Kitchen Pharmacy*, Orion Books, London, 1998

Family Guide to Alternative Medicine, Reader's Digest Association, London, 1991

Flanagan, Sabina, *Hildegard of Bingen: A Visionary Life*, Routledge, London, 1998

Fowler, Deborah, *Nature's Pharmacy*, Truran Books, Truro, 2004

Fowler, Deborah, and Cuckson, Sally, *The Herb Book*, Truran Books, Truro, 2003

Gray, Linda, *Traditional Remedies*, Ebury Press, London, 2007

Grieve, Mrs M., *A Modern Herbal*, Jonathan Cape, London, 1931 (reprinted Penguin Books, Harmondsworth, 1976)

Hatfield, Gabrielle, *Memory, Wisdom and Healing*, Sutton Publishing Ltd, Stroud, 2005

Hunt, Rachel, *The Wholefood Harvest Cookbook: Gourmet Recipes from Garden to Table*, Gallery Books, London, 1990

Kennett, Frances, *Folk Medicine: Fact and Fiction*, Marshall Cavendish, London, 1984

Kirk, E.W., *Tried Favourites Cookery Book: With Household Hints and Other Useful Information*, A.D. Johnston, Edinburgh, 1948

Kirkpatrick, Betty, *Auld Scottish Grannies' Remedies*, Crombie Jardine Publishing Ltd, Bath, 2005

Le Fanu, James, *The Daily Telegraph Complete Home Remedies*, Robinson, London, 1999

Mabey, Richard, *Food for Free: A Guide to the Edible Wild Plants of Britain*, William Collins Sons & Co Ltd, 1972

McIntyre, Anne, *The Complete Floral Healer: The Healing Power of Flowers through Herbalism, Aromatherapy and Homeopathy*, Gaia Books Ltd, London, 2002

McIntyre, Anne, *Healing Drinks: Juices, Teas, Soups, Smoothies*, Gaia Books Ltd, London, 2004

McIntyre, Anne, *Herbal Treatment of Children*, Elsevier Health Sciences, London, 2005

Metcalfe, Joannah, *Herbs and Aromatherapy*, Bloomsbury Books, London, 1992

Moody, Joanna (ed.), *Private Life of an Elizabethan Lady: The Diary of Lady Margaret Hoby* 1599–1605, Sutton Publishing Ltd, Stroud, 1998

Plowden, Alison, *Elizabethan England: Life in an Age of Invention*, Reader's Digest Association, London, 1982

Pole, Sebastian, *Ayurvedic Medicine: The Principles of Traditional Practice*, Churchill Livingstone, Elsevier, London, 2006

Rappaport, Helen, *No Place for Ladies: The Untold Story of Women in the Crimean War*, Aurum Press, London, 2007

Reid, Daniel P., *The Tao of Health, Sex and Longevity: A Modern Practical Guide to the Ancient Way*, Simon & Schuster, New York, 1989

Rousselet-Blanc, Josette and Vincent, *Les remèdes de grand-mères*, Éditions Michel Lafon, Neuilly-sur-Seine, 2001

Seacole, Mary, *Wonderful Adventures of Mrs Seacole in Many Lands*, 1857 (reprinted Oxford University Press, Oxford, 1988)

Stewart, Maryon, *The Natural Menopause Kit: Beat Menopause Naturally and be Yourself Again*, Vine House Distribution, 2007

Tusser, Thomas, *Five Hundred Points of Good Husbandry*, 1557 (reprinted Oxford University Press, Oxford, 1984)

Van Straten, Michael, and Griggs, Barbara, *Superfoods*, Dorling Kindersley, London, 1990

Vaughan, J.G. and Judd, P.A., *The Oxford Book of Health Foods*, Oxford University Press, Oxford, 2003

Zaczek, Iain, *Chronicles of the Celts*, Collins & Brown, London, 1996

Acknowledgements

I am immensely grateful to the many marvellous members of the Women's Institute and the readers of *Saga Magazine* and *Scots Magazine*, who offered their own and their families' remedies. Catherine Gould, Hazel Townesend and Anne Bisset also contributed copies of their grandmothers' and great-grandmothers' handwritten books of 'receipts', which provided a fascinating insight to their lives, and Colin McLeod and Margaret Smith provided original handwritten remedies.

Special thanks also go to: Andie Airfix of Satori; Carola Augustin; Marina Augustin; Richard Bailey; Jackie Bean; Pauline Chatterley; Dee Cook, archivist of the Worshipful Society of the Apothecaries of London; the late Peter Cooper and his family; Jo Cumming of Arthritis Care; Ian Varney Fenton; Deborah Fowler of Halzephron Herb Farm; Peter Homan and Briony Hudson of the Royal Pharmaceutical Society of Great Britain; Penny Kitchen of WI Publications; Sophie Lazar of Random House Publishing; Anne McIntyre; Laura Morris; Dr Henry Oakeley FRCP and the Royal College of Physicians; David Orr; Martine Pey of Vienna; Sebastian Pole; Powys County Archives Office; Helen Rappaport; Professor Nick Read, medical adviser of the Gut Trust; Patrick Swan; Roger Tabor, past president of the Herb Society; and the Rev. Canon Celia Thomson.

Every effort has been made to contact all copyright holders. If notified, we will be pleased to rectify any errors or omissions at the earliest opportunity.

Index

Cook, Captain, 198
Cookworthy, William, 90
Cooper, Peter, 77, 134
Coppen-Gardner, Sylvia, 60
copper bracelets, 128
coriander (*Coriandrum sativum*), 89, 137, *137*
corns, 52–3
Costley, Sarah, 124
Coton Manor Garden, 232
cotton wool, burned, 60
coughs, 53–8
cracked heels, 58
Crete, 34
Crimean War, 199, 200–1
Cross, Katherine, 146
Crossley, Jean, 46
Cruces, Panama, 199–200
cucumber, 138
Culpeper, Nicholas, 5, 22–3, 54–5, 101, 117, 148, 149, 155–6, 174, 190–1, 193–6, 196–7
Culpeper shops, 175, 202
Cumming, Jo, 126–7
curry, 46
curry plant (*Helichrysum italicum*), 217
cuts
    minor, 58–60
    serious or infected, 60–2
Cymbopogon citratus, see citronella
cypress, 63

dandelions (*Taraxacum officinalis*), 2, 16, 83, 110–11, *111*, 163–4, 165, *165*, 195–6, 207, 211, 218

dandruff, 63–4
Darius the Great, 9
Dark Ages, 172
Darlington, Dr Gail, 132, 134
Davies, Anna, 40, 80–1, 112, 150
Davison, Pam, 138–9
decoctions, making, 223–4
depression, 64–6
dermatitis, 66–7
detoxification, 67–71
Devereux, Robert, Earl of Essex, 187
Devereux, Walter, 187
Devon WI, 19, 55, 88
diarrhoea, 71–3
Dickens, Charles, 17
dill, 43
Diocletian, emperor, 177
Dioscorides, 21, 196
Dipsacus fullonum, see teasles
Disibodenberg, 182
dock (*Rumex*), 120
Doctrine of Signatures, 194–6, 197
dog bites, 73–4
Dolly Blue, 15
Donaghue, Pam, 41
Droitwich Spa Lido, 232
Drysdale, Norman, 18, 208
dulse, 52
dyer's greenweed (*Genista tinctoria*), 217
dyer's madder (*Rubia tinctorum*), 217
dysentery, 72, 186

earache, 75–6
ears, *see* earache; tinnitus

eau-de-Cologne, 13
eels, 59
eggs, 3, 49, 72, 91, 95, 134, *151*, 167
    white, 3, 14, 25, 123, 140–1, 151–2, 158
    yolk, 25, 48, 111, 150
Egyptians, 87, 100, 122, 148, 171–2
Einion, 181
elder (*Sambucus*), 140, 155–6
    berries, 57, *57*
    flowers, 13, 19–20, *20*, 39–40, 77, 147
Eleanor of Aquitaine, 172–3
Elizabeth I, Queen, 187, 190
Elliot, Rose, 46, 86, 88
Elliott, Lily, 129–30
elm, slippery (*Ulmus rubra*), 62, 103–4, 228
Englishman's Doctor, The, 84
Epstein, Jacob, 210
Essex, Robert Devereux, Earl of, 187
Eton, 191
eucalyptus, 21, 37–8, *38*, 93
Eupatorium cannabinum, see hemp agrimony
Euphrasia officinalis, see eyebright
evening primroses (*Oenothera*), 218
exercise, 128
eyebright (*Euphrasia officinalis*), 195
eyes
    sight deficiencies, 123–4
    tired and sore, 76–7
    see also styes

glycyrrhizin, 22, 149
goldenrod (*Solidago*), 195–6
goldenseal (*Hydrastis canadensis*), 11
Goodman, Marjorie, 17
Goodson, Mary, 12
goose fat, 21
Görlitz, 195
goulard water, 146
Gould, Catherine, 13, 26, 48, 145
gout, 85–7
Gray, Linda, 98, 102, 117
grazes, 87
grease, 21
Great Rissington, 211–12
Greece, 177, 178
Greeks, Ancient, 58, 65, 68, 100, 148, 172
Grieve, Mrs, 1, 8, 19, 22, 39–40, 50, 57, 61, 82, 111, 136, 140, 151, 165, 168, 175, 202–3
Griffiths, Joan, 45, 142
Griggs, Barbara, 16, 86
gripe water, 43
Gruffud, 181
Guatemala, 69
Guild of Structural Integration, 205
Gut Trust, 103
gynaecology, 179–80

Hackness estate, 187, 188, 190
haemorrhoids, 88–9
halitosis, 89
Hamamelis, see witch hazel
Han dynasty, 22

hands
  cold and chapped, 34–5
  sweaty, 147
hangover, 90–1
Hanna, Maureen, 52
Harper Deacon, Jennifer, 163
Harry, Richard, 163
hartshorn, 51, 78, 135
harvesting, 219–20
Hatcher, Julia, 129
Hatshepsut, 171
Hawkins, Barbara, 23
Hawkins, Cynthia, 102
hayfever, 92
head lice, 94–6
headache, 92–3
heat, 12
Helianthus, see sunflower
Helichrysum italicum, see curry plant
Helpman, Robert, 133
hemp agrimony (*Eupatorium cannabinum*), 8, 11, 217
Henry IV, King of France, 187
herbal myths, ix–xi
herbs
  drying and storing, 220–2
  harvesting, 219–20
  preparing for use, 222–9
  selecting, 217–18
  starting a garden, 215–16
  see also names of herbs
Herb Society (formerly Society of Herbalists), 175, 202
Hewitt, Mrs, 88
Hezekiah, 1

hiccups, 96
Hildegard of Bingen, 47, 66, 92, 136, 173, 182–6
Hilton, Mary, 59
Hippocrates, xii, 16, 32, 47, 48, 62, 68, 107, 140
Hoby, Lady Margaret, 186–91
Hoby, Sir Thomas, 188
Homan, Peter, 14, 26, 135
Home & Country, 39, 42, 55, 98, 105, 120, 208
honey
  for acne, 2
  for ageing, 4
  for burns, 24
  for chapped hands, 34
  for chills, 30
  for cold sores, 36
  for colds, 38, 40, 41
  for coughs, 55, 56, 57
  for earache, 75
  for hayfever, 92
  for indigestion, 102
  for sore throats, 211
  for whooping cough, 167
  used for making syrup, 225
  used as poultice, 228
Hopper, Mrs E.C., 19
hops (*Humulus*), 108, *108*
hormone replacement therapy, 116
Horrocks, Samuel Thornley, 41
horse chestnuts, 207, 208
horseradish (*Armoracia rusticana*), 219
hot flushes, 114–15

lead acetate, 33, 146
lectucarium, 106–7
leeks, 86, 117
lemon, 154
  barley water recipe, 113–14
  for chills, 30
  for colds, 41
  for convalescence, 49
  for coughs, 56
  for diarrhoea, 72
  for halitosis, 89
  for head lice and nits, 95
  for indigestion, 101, 102, 103
  for liver complaints, 110
  for tonsillitis, 154
  for warts, 164
lemon balm, 121
lemon grass (citronella; *Cymbopogon citratus*), 105
lemon verbena (*Aloysia triphylla*), 27, 138
lettuce, 106–7
Leucozade, 207
Levisticum officinale, see lovage
Leyel, Hilda, 175, 202–3
lily leaves, 60
lime (calcium hydroxide), 26
lime (*Tilia*)
  blossom/flowers, 108, 108, 144
  juice, 115
liniments, making, 227
Linnaeus, 86
lin, seed (flax; *Linum usitatissimum*), 61
  oil, 26

Linton, Yorkshire, 187
Linum usitatissimum, see lin, seed
lipoproteins, 34
liquorice (*Glycyrrhiza glabra*), 21–2, 45, 52, 121, 149
Littleton WI, 27, 59, 93
liver complaints, 110–11
lobelia oil, 141
London, 190, 192, 194, 197, 199, 201
London School of Medicine for Women, 197
Loseley Park, 233
lovage (*Levisticum officinale*), 116, 216, 217
Love's Labour's Lost, 22
Lowther, Nancy, 21
lungwort (*Pulmonaria*), 195
Lynas, Margaret, 162

Maby, Richard, 91
McCartney, Sir Paul, 210
McElhinney, May, 112
McElhinney, Robert, 20, 45, 52, 94
McIntyre, Anne, 39, 99, 104, 137, 144–5, 159–60, 211–14, 224
Mckenzie, John, 160
Mclay, Sheena, 139
McLeod, Colin, 134
'magnetic' bracelets, 128
maidenhair fern (*Adiantum capillus-veneris*), 196
mallow (*Malva*), 27, 92, 138, 138
malt extract, 98

Malva, see mallow
Manitoba, 7
marigolds, pot (*Calendula officinalis*), 5, 10–11, 19, 112, 115, 145, 195–6, 217, 218, 221–2
marjoram (*Origanum*), 4, 5, 29, 217, 218
marshmallow (*Althaea officinalis*), 104, 112, 217
marsh trefoil (*Menyanthes trifoliata*; bog bean; buckbean), 20
Martin, Dr Vivien, 135, 151
Martindale's Pharmacopoeia, 32
massage, 5–6, 7, 11, 12–13, 93, 112, 129
mastitis, 112
match heads, 164
Mead, Janet, 10, 138
meadowsweet (*Filipendula ulmaria*), 217
measles, 112–14
meat tenderiser, 109
Mediterranean diet, 34
melissa, 93
Melville, Marjorie, 51, 63, 130
menopause, 114–16
menstruation, 116–17
Mentha, see mint
  piperita, see peppermint
Menyanthes trifoliata (bog bean; buckbean; marsh trefoil), 20
mercury, 32, 33, 175
Metcalfe, Joannah, 95
methylated spirits, 13–14, 134

sorrel, 111, 221
South Africa, 109, 206
South America, xi, 198
Southampton, University of, 17
southernwood (*Artemisia abrotanum*), 217–18
Spencer, Mrs, 55
spermacetti, 34
Spero, Di, 153
sphagnum moss (*Sphagnum cymbilofolium*), 61–2, 207
spiders' webs, 58–9, *59*, 62
Spitalfields, 194
splinters, 138–9
sprains, 140–1
spring onions, 120
springs, 123–4
starch, 35
steam, 3, 37–8, 42, 69, 70, 139
   baths, 69
Stellaria media, *see* chickweed
Stewart, Maryon, 115
stiff necks, 142
Stobart, Anne, 29–30, 56
Straten, Michael van, 16 19, 86
strawberries, 86
stress, 142–5
stroke, 45
Stubbins, Janet, 129, 145
styes, 145–6
sugar
   for acne, 3
   for anxiety, 6
   for diarrhoea, 73

for hiccups, 96
for splinter removal, 138–9
   making syrup, 225–6
used as ingredient in remedies, 1, 8, 40, 48, 55, 56, 57, 58, 71, 72, 97, 101, 102, 119, 150, 152, 158, 167
Sulgrave Manor, 235
sulphur, 17, 63, 70–1, 164
sunburn, 146–7
Sunday Times, 163
sunflower (*Helianthus*), 218
   oil, 226
Sung Dynasty, 68
superstition, xiv, 172
surgical spirit, 135
sweat lodges, 69
sweating regimes, 69–71
sweating sickness, 186–7
sweaty hands and feet, 147
Sweden, 198
swedes, 55
Swift, Cynthia, 120, 149, 159
Swiss, the, 110
Swiss Technical University, 204
sweet cicely (*Myrrhis odorata*), 217, 218
swollen glands, 142
Symphytum, *see* comfrey
syrups, making, 225–6

Tanacetum, *see* tansy *parthenium*, *see* feverfew
tansy (*Tanacetum*), *100*, 101
tar, 41
Taraxacum officinale, *see* dandelions

tarragon, 221
tartar, 167
tea, 72, 77, 79, 85, 147, 211
   herbal, *see* infusions, making
tea-tree, 95, 122
teasles (*Dipsacus fullonum*), 217
teeth cleaning, 148–9
thistle, milk (*Silybum marianum*), 90–1, *91*, 196
Thomson, Rev. Canon Celia, 119
Thomson, Marie, 132–3
throats, sore, 149–52
thyme (*Thymus*), 61, 62, 79–80, *80*, 89, 104, 121, 168, 218, 221–2
ticks, 152
Tilia, *see* lime
Timms, Margaret, 96
tinctures, making, 224–5
tinnitus, 153
tobacco, 166
toddy, 29–30
toenails, 153–4
tonsillitis, 154–5
toothache, 155–6
toothpaste, 4, 36
toothpicks, 149
Townesend, Gwladys, 139
Townesend, Hazel, 139
Townsend, Judy, 3, 38, 143
Tramaseur, Dru, 153
travel sickness, 157
treacle, 17–18, 41, 54
Trifolium pratense, *see* clover, red
Trinity Hall, Cambridge, 191